Weight Watchers

Get Ready For 2018 With The Complete Smart Points Guide to A Permanent Weight Lost Include 90 Day Meal Plan

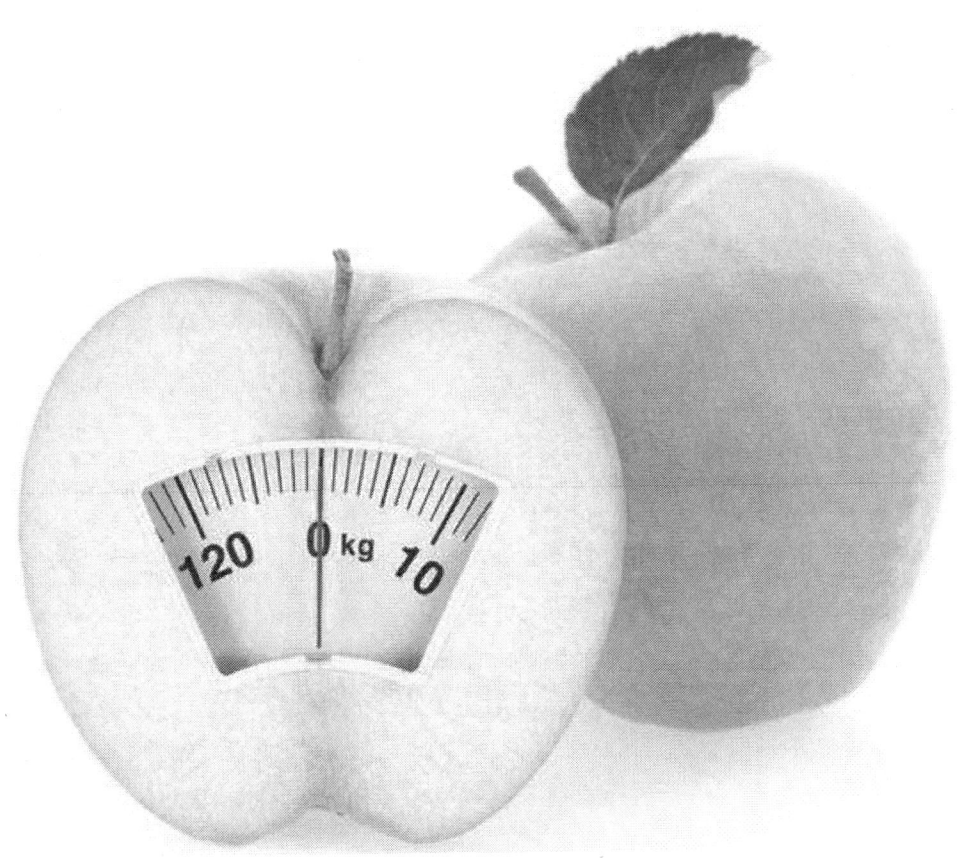

By Lara Croft

Copyright 2017 by Lara Croft. All rights reserved.

This document is geared towards providing exact and reliable information in regards to the topic and issue covered. The publication is sold with the idea that the publisher is not required to render accounting, officially permitted, or otherwise, qualified services. If advice is necessary, legal or professional, a practiced individual in the profession should be ordered.

- From a Declaration of Principles which was accepted and approved equally by a Committee of the American Bar Association and a Committee of Publishers and Associations.

In no way is it legal to reproduce, duplicate, or transmit any part of this document in either electronic means or in printed format. Recording of this publication is strictly prohibited and any storage of this document is not allowed unless with written permission from the publisher. All rights reserved.

The information provided herein is stated to be truthful and consistent, in that any liability, in terms of inattention or otherwise, by any usage or abuse of any policies, processes, or directions contained within is the solitary and utter responsibility of the recipient reader. Under no circumstances will any legal responsibility or blame be held against the publisher for any reparation, damages, or monetary loss due to the information herein, either directly or indirectly.

Respective authors own all copyrights not held by the publisher.

The information herein is offered for informational purposes solely, and is universal as so. The presentation of the information is without contract or any type of guarantee assurance.

The trademarks that are used are without any consent, and the publication of the trademark is without permission or backing by the trademark owner. All trademarks and brands within this book are for clarifying purposes only and are the owned by the owners themselves, not affiliated with this document.

Disclaimer: This book is for informational purposes only. Use of the guidelines in this book is a choice of the reader. This book is not intended for the treatment or prevention of disease. This book is also, not a substitute for medical treatment or an alternative to medical advice.

Table of Contents

Weight Watchers and Smart Points 7

How Does It Work 9

Breakfast Recipes 18

    Mediterranean Strata with Goat Cheese 19

    Cheesy and Saucy Egg Sandwich 20

    Hash and Eggs 21

    Creamy Scrambled Eggs with Scallions and Tomatoes 22

    Steak and Eggs 23

    Passion Fruit Soufflé Omelette and Blueberries 24

    Mexican Breakfast Burritos 25

Egg, Canadian Bacon, Avocado, and Tomato Sandwich 26
Mini Zucchini Quiche 27
Italian Pepper and Egg Sandwich 28
Fluffy Lemon-Ricotta Pancakes 29
Quinoa and Apple Breakfast Cereal 30
Whole-Grain Banana Pancakes with Blackberry Syrup 31
Cheesy Vegetable Sandwich 32
French Toast Nuggets 33
Oat and Apricot Bars 34
Bacon, Egg, and Spinach Stacks 35
Chicken BLT Sandwich 36
Denver Omelette in a Mug 37

Pork Recipes 38
Spice-Rubbed Pork Chops 39
Pork Tenderloin Roast 40
Seasoned Pork Tenderloin 41
Roast Pork Dinner 42
Cider-Glazed Pork Chops with Apples and Cabbage 43
Pulled Pork Special 44
Sesame-Ginger Pork Tenderloin 45
Breaded Pork Cutlet 46
Spicy Asian Pork Tenderloin 47
Bacon-Bundled BBQ Shrimp 49

Beef Recipes 50
Roasted Sirloin Beef 51
Filet Mignon with Red Wine Sauce 52
Buffalo Ranch Meatloaf 53
Bacon Cheeseburger Chili 54
100-Calorie Beef Patties 55
Stir-Fry Beef and Broccoli 56
Steak and Mushroom with Mashies 57
Amazing Cheeseburger Patty 58

Chicken Recipes 59

- Baked Chicken 60
- Feta-Stuffed Chicken Burgers 61
- General Tso's Chicken 62
- Italian Pesto Chicken Burger 63
- Taco Stuffed Chicken 64
- Spinach and Feta Stuffed Chicken 65
- Kickin' Chicken Pot Pie 66
- Fajita-Stuffed Chicken 67
- Tandoori Chicken with Chutney 68
- Chinese Chicken Salad 70
- BBQ Chicken Quesadilla 71

Fish Recipes 72
- Roasted Salmon in Honey-Mustard 73
- Spicy BBQ Salmon and Veggies 74
- Grilled Salmon with Mustard 75
- Grilled Yellowfin Tuna with Teriyaki Sauce 76
- Grilled Fish with Tartar Sauce 77
- Grilled Trout with Stuffed Oregano and Lemon 78

Vegetable Recipes 79
- Barley-Asparagus Risotto with Balsamic Vinegar ... 80
- Baked Vegetable Tart 81
- Cellophane Noodles with Garlic, Cilantro, and Cucumbers ... 82
- Grilled BBQ Tempeh 83
- Bok Choy and Tofu Stir-Fry 84
- California Club Wrap 85
- Greek-Style Spaghetti Squash 86
- Tomato-Basil Sauce Eggplant Involtini 87
- Grilled Vegetables and Haloumi 89
- Artichoke and Red Pepper Frittata 90
- Eggplant Parmigiana 91
- Caramelized Onion and Mushroom Lasagna 92
- Baked Pasta with Butternut Squash 94
- Chickpea and Brown Rice Veggie Burgers with Tomato Salad ... 95

Soup Recipes ... 97
- Zero Hero Soup ... 98
- Cream of Broccoli Soup ... 99
- Italian-Inspired Vegetable Soup ... 100
- Super Easy Chicken Noodle Soup ... 101
- Veggie Soup ... 102
- Fresh Vegetable Soup ... 103
- Beef, Mushroom, and Barley Soup ... 104
- Garden Vegetable Soup ... 105
- Chicken and Root Vegetables Soup ... 106

Dessert Recipes ... 107
- Ultimate Fruit Salad ... 108
- Crunchy Chocolate Mousse with Strawberries ... 109
- Ricotta and Almond Stuffed Dates ... 110
- Grilled Mango with Raspberry Granita ... 111
- Blueberry Pie ... 112
- Peaches and Cream Tart ... 113
- Baby Chocolate Butterfly Cakes ... 114
- Apricot Dessert Quesadillas ... 115
- Spiced Turkish Mocha ... 116

Snack Recipes ... 117
- Fruit Salad with Spiced Pistachio Yoghurt ... 118
- Sultana and Apple Slice ... 119
- Strawberry and Blueberry Muffins ... 120
- Berry Bliss Balls ... 121
- Cauliflower, Mint, and Feta Fritters ... 122
- Bacon Bundled Asparagus ... 123
- Spicy Popcorn ... 124
- Coconut and Date Muesli Bars ... 125
- Pepper and Mushroom Kebabs with Dip ... 126
- Lemon-Rosemary White Bean Bruschetta ... 127
- Buffalo-Style Stuffed Celery ... 128
- Butternut Squash Fries ... 129

- Chocolate-Banana Mini Muffins 130
- Roasted Cauliflower with Lemon and Garlic 131
- Maple Granola Bars 132

Slow Cook Recipes 133
- Crock Pot Loaded Beef Stew: 134
- Thai Chicken Soup: 136
- Tasty Bourbon Chicken: 137
- Protein Chicken Tacos: 138
- Sweet Potato Chili: 139
- One Pot Pumpkin Chili: 140
- Apple Butter Pulled Pork: 141
- Bean and Potato Soup: 142
- White Bean and Chicken Chili: 143
- Chicken and Rice Casserole: 144
- Honey Mustard Chicken: 145
- Loaded Creamy Corn Chowder: 146
- Chunky Squash & Chicken Stew: 147
- Cauliflower Fried Rice: 148

The Ultimate 3-Month Meal Plan 148

Conclusion 167

Introduction

This book covers the topic of Smart Points and the Weight Watchers diet and will teach you how to achieve a healthy and fit body without exerting too much effort.

This book contains recipes plus other food combinations that you can mix and match. It includes a 3-month meal plan so you don't need to worry so much about what to eat for the day.

At the completion of this book, you will have a good understanding of the Smart Points system and do the things that you must do –without cheating. You may even get to prepare your own dish and determine its Smart Points!

Weight Watchers and Smart Points

Weight Watchers is an American company founded on May 15, 1963. It offers numerous products and services that aim to help you maintain your ideal weight or lose some pounds. When you hear a discussion involving Weight Watchers, you will also hear about Smart Points.

What are Smart Points?

Smart Points is actually a counting system that was made popular by Weight Watchers. It can help you choose the right foods to consume within the day without making you feel sluggish and hungry. You will eat, feel, and look better than before you have decided to get into the program. You will lose weight and gain more energy. You will definitely increase your productivity and gain more time to spend with family and friends.

In rating the different foods, those with high sugar content and/or saturated fat have high Smart Points. The foods with high amount of lean protein have lower Smart Points.

Keep these in Mind when dealing with Smart Points

1. Every food has its own Smart Points value, which is calculated based on the amount of sugar, saturated fat, calories, and protein.

2. Protein can lower the Smart Points of the food (the lower the Smart Points of the food, the better).

3. Saturated fats and sugar can increase the Smart Points value of the food.

Weight Watchers Benefits

Researchers from Germany, Australia, and the UK found that the patients who were recommended by their doctors to follow the Weight Watchers program lost about twice as much weight as compared to those who chose the usual weight loss program. The findings were reported in The Lancet.

The American Journal of Lifestyle Medicine also published a study regarding the 6-month long Weight Watchers group program. The obese or overweight adults who diligently attended the two-thirds of the sessions on a weekly basis have diminished some weight and their insulin and glucose levels have been radically reduced.

In Chapter 3, you will see a list of the different foods that most people consume daily plus the Smart Points value of each food. If you have no time to prepare or you can't decide what to eat, you can refer to the chart for a quick fix. However, it is still best to follow a meal plan.

Don't make it a habit to always peek on the chart and be contented with the quick fixes to satisfy your hunger.

The next section contain different recipes, aside from the food list, that are included in the 3-month meal plan in the end of the book. When you have decided to create your own meal plan, you can whip your own or include the recipes from the said section.

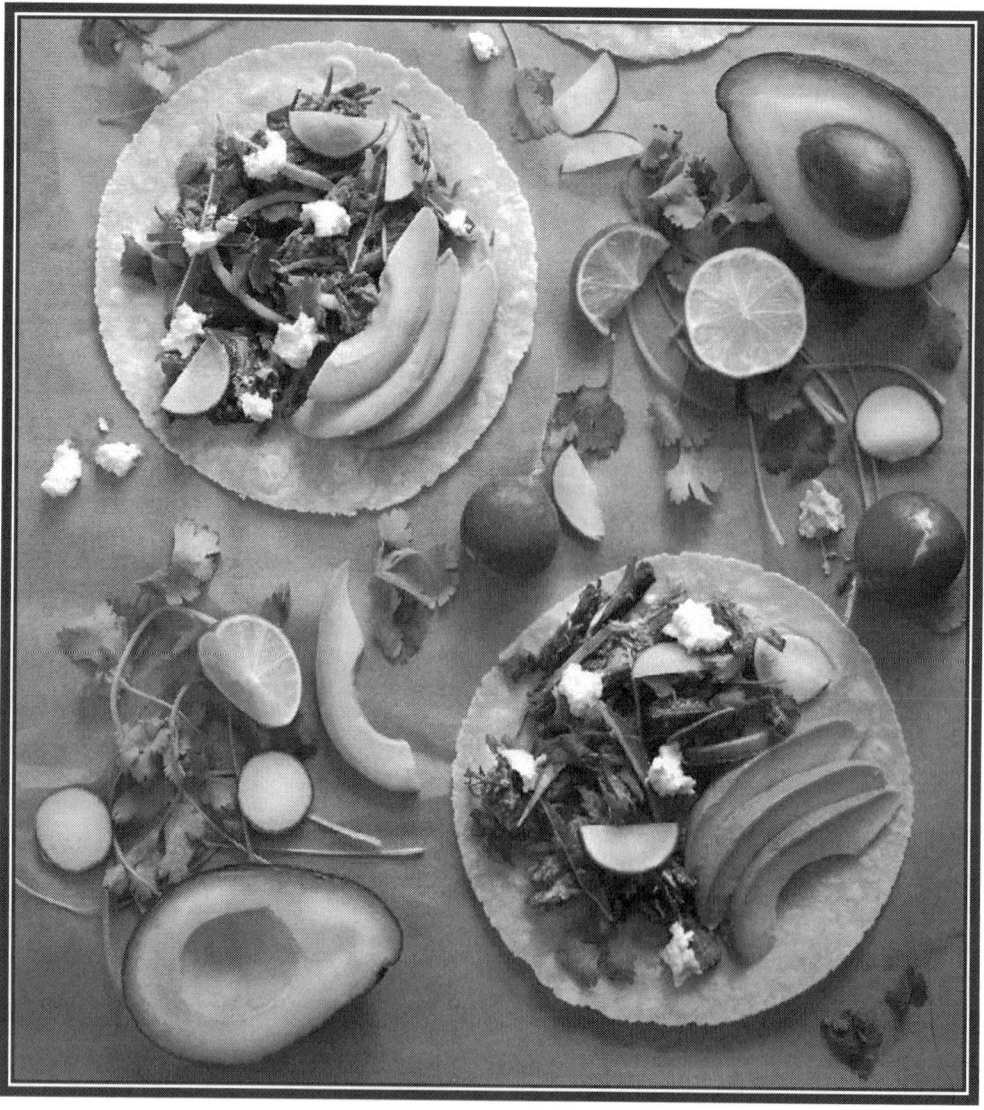

How Does It Work

When you have decided to follow the Weight Watchers 'way of attaining an ideal body weight, then you must know the daily Smart Points that you are allowed to spend. There is a formula that can help you compute your daily Smart Points allowance or you can go to this online calculator:

http://www.healthyweightforum.org/eng/calculators/ww-points-allowed/

The online calculator can give you the daily Smart Points that you are only allowed to spend per week so you can achieve your ideal weight. It also gives the number of weeks that it would take before you see the expected result. Although it is important to strictly adhere to your daily Smart Points allowance, you are also given a weekly allowance of 35 flexible Smart Points that you can spend to gain bigger allowance or when you need to dine out.

You must have noticed that the level of activity is included in computing the daily Smart Points that you are allowed to spend. When you enter the data being asked, provide your current level of activity. You can choose to do simple exercises while spending the suggested Smart Points that you are permitted to spend.

You can get extra fit points (when you do additional activity) if you enroll in the Weight Watchers program. After achieving your weight goal, you can re-calculate your daily Smart Points and you can enter your new level of activity.

The Activity Levels

The online calculator presents four activity levels:

1. The Sedentary Level

Your activity level is sedentary if you sit most of the day in the office or at home. You may also have a bit of slow walking and do light household chores that can be accomplished in minutes.

2. Light Level

You have a light activity level if you do the things in the sedentary level plus other activities that usually take 2 hours to accomplish. It could be brisk walking, gardening, and/or heavy housework.

3. Moderate Level

In the moderate level, you may still be doing the things in light level but occasional walking is obvious. You engage in a vigorous exercise such as swimming and dancing. There's no trace of sedentary life in your daily activity and you can move swiftly.

4. High or Heavy

If you have high levels of activity, you are always on the go. You don't let yourself get idle and slack off. However, it is also important to keep in mind that a little rest is also good for the body. Don't abuse your body with too much activity.

Smart Points of a Particular Food

Each food has their corresponding Smart Points value. Your choice of food depends on the daily Smart Points allowance that you are allowed to spend. You cannot go beyond the set limit to make the program work for you. In this regard, proper meal planning is truly necessary. If you will not follow the requirement, then don't expect to see a favorable result. You only get yourself to blame.

There is also a formula that can help compute the Smart Points value of each food, but it is still best to go to this online calculator to see the Smart Points value of each food:

http://www.exercise4weightloss.com/smart-points-calculator.html

In using the online Smart Points value calculator, you need to provide the calorie, sugar, protein, and fat content of a particular food that you intend to eat (in case it is something out of your usual set of fares).

A Glimpse of the Weight Watchers Points System

To give you some background regarding the point system, in case you want to compute manually, you can use this formula:

$$SP = \frac{calories}{33} + \frac{saturated\ fat}{4} + \frac{sugar}{8} - \frac{protein}{10}$$

You need to round off the result to get the Smart Points value of a particular food.

The foods that are low in fat and/or have high fiber content are usually worth fewer points. This only means that you can eat more of these foods than fares with high points. If you have low Smart Points allowance to spend, then you can only consume large amounts of foods with low Smart Points value.

To know your Smart Points allowance per day, look at this chart as a guide:

If you are:	The Equivalent Points
Female	2
Nursing Female	10
Male	8
between 16 and 17 years old	4
between 27 and 37 years old	3
between 38 and 47 years old	2
between 48 and 57 years old	1
between 58 and older	0
exercising every day for more than 30 minutes or doing manual labor	6
exercising every day for more than 30 minutes or walking in your workplace	4
standing or moving most of the time	2
living a sedentary life	0
between 155cm and shorter	0
between 155cm and 178cm	1
between 178cm and above	2
*get the 10% of your weight in pounds	the result will serve as your points

After getting the corresponding points, you need to get the sum of your points and that would be your Smart Points allowance. Please take note that the chart does not give any time frame when you could see visible results, unlike the online calculator.

Important Things to Remember About the Points

1. You cannot roll over the unused daily Smart Points allowance and flexible points to the following day and week. The unused points will be lost and can no longer be exhausted.

2. It is important to drink lots of water because it can help your body flush toxins out. Also, drinking plenty of water can help keep you feel full for a long time. You need to drink more if you are working out to keep your body hydrated.

3. It is recommended to at least include simple exercise routines to get your body moving. You will also feel light and nimble when you exercise.

4. Choose a nutritious meal, regardless of the Smart Points value of the foods. The lean meats and fresh, organic vegetables can give you a fit and healthy body for a long time.

5. Most fruits and vegetables have 0 points value, so it is safe to consume more of them in case you need to eat extra.

Don't hesitate to use your flexible points if you need more food, especially when you have more workload than usual. Do not starve yourself. There are plenty of foods that have 0 point value.

Spending your Smart Points

You already know about the points and how to get your daily Smart Points allowance. Now, you are ready to spend your Smart Points allowance.

If your daily Smart Points allowance is 30, then you should not eat beyond your limit. However, you can always use your flexible points (more about it later). For example, you want an egg, some bacon, cheese, and spinach with olive oil. Understand that the 30 Smart Points allowance is good for one day, which includes 3 meals and 2 snacks.

A whole egg is worth 2 points. The 2 oz. chopped Canadian bacon is worth 2 points. The 2 tablespoons low-fat shredded cheddar cheese is worth 1 point. The spinach and onion are worth 0 points. The 1 teaspoon olive oil is worth 1 point. When you tally the points, you will get a total of 6 points. If you want to add chopped tomatoes and/or fresh herbs, you will still get 6 points. It is because the things that you want to add are all worth 0 points. You still have 24 Smart Points that you can spend for the remaining meals of the day.

Things you need to keep in Mind

Your daily Smart Points allowance is personalized to you. It is really up to you how to use or distribute it. You can also follow this sample distribution table:

Daily Allowance	30	35	40	45	50	55	60	65	70
Breakfast	6	7	8	8	9	9	10	11	12
Snack	3	4	4	5	5	6	6	7	8
Lunch	8	9	10	12	14	16	17	18	20
Snack	2	3	3	4	4	4	5	5	6
Dinner	11	12	15	16	18	20	22	24	24

To get more from your daily allowance, you need to target the foods with smaller Smart Points value. If you need to adjust (increase your intake using your flexible points), it is best to make adjustments on your snacks.

As you make progress, your target will definitely change. In the provided online calculator for your daily Smart Points allowance, you will notice that there are weeks when you have lower points allowance to spend.

You can also consult your doctor and ask if you need to follow certain protocol in your diet. You can also ask for some vitamin-mineral supplements that you can take along with your diet.

You need to be kind to yourself. Make healthy choices, follow your budget, and don't stop halfway. Remember that this endeavor is not a temporary fix–you are actually changing your lifestyle into a better one.

List of Most Tracked Foods

Below is the table of most tracked foods (and some more) together with their Smart Points value:

Most Tracked Foods	Smart Points Value
Almond milk: 1 cup: unsweetened: plain	1
Almonds: 1/4 cup	4
American cheese: 1oz or 1 slice	4
Apple	0
Asparagus	0
Avocado : 1/4	2
Bacon : 3 slices : cooked	5
Bagel of any type: 2oz: 1/2 large or 1 small	5
Banana	0
Beef : 3oz : 90% lean : ground : cooked	4
Beer: 12oz: regular	5
Berries: mixed	0
Black beans: 1/2 cup: canned	3
Blackberries	0

Food	Value
Blueberries	0
Bread : 1 slice	2
Broccoli	0
Brown rice: 1 cup: cooked	6
Butter: 1 tablespoon	5
Cantaloupe	0
Carrots	0
Carrots: baby	0
Celery	0
Cheddar cheese: 1/4 cup: shredded	4
Cheddar cheese: 2 tbsps.: shredded: low fat	1
Cheddar or Colby cheese : 1oz	4
Cherries	0
Cherry tomatoes	0
Chicken breast : 3oz : skinless : cooked : boneless	2
Coffee : black : 1 cup	0
Cookies : 1 or 1/2oz : homemade : chocolate chip : oatmeal : sugar : other similar types	3
Corn on the cob : 1 medium	4
Cottage cheese : 1 cup : fat-free	2
Cream: 2 tbsps.: half and half	2
Cucumber	0
Deli sliced turkey : 2oz	1
Diet Coke: 8oz	0
Egg white : 1	0
Egg: 1 whole	2
Egg: 1 whole: fried	3
Eggs: 2: scrambled with milk and butter	6
English muffin: 1 or 2oz	4
Feta : 1oz : crumbled	3
French fries: 5.5oz	13
Fruit: unsweetened: fresh	0
Grape tomatoes	0
Grapefruit	0
Grapes	0
Green beans	0
Guacamole: 2 tbsps.	1

Item	Points
Half and half: 2 tbsps.: fat-free	1
Hamburger bun: 1 or 2oz: plain	5
Honey: 1 tbsp.	4
Hummus: 2 tbsps.	2
Lettuce	0
Luncheon meat : 2oz : lean : ham : honey : deli-sliced	2
Mango	0
Mashed potatoes: 1/2 cup	4
Mayonnaise : 1 tablespoon	3
Milk: 1 cup: low fat 1%	4
Milk: 1 cup: reduced fat 2%	5
Milk: 1 cup: skim (fat-free)	3
Milk: 1 cup: whole	7
Mushrooms	0
Mustard: 1 tbsp.	0
Nectarine	0
Oatmeal: 1 cup: cooked	1
Olive oil: 1 tbsp.	4
Onions	0
Orange	0
Pasta: 1 cup: cooked: regular or whole wheat	5
Peach	0
Peanut butter: 2 tbsps.	6
Pear	0
Pineapple	0
Pork chop : 3oz : lean : cooked : boneless	3
Potato : 1.6oz : plain : baked	5
Raspberries	0
Red wine: 5oz	4
Salad dressing : 1 tbsp. : low-fat : balsamic vinaigrette	1
Salad dressing: 2 tbsps. : Italian-type (not creamy)	3
Salad dressing: 2 tbsps.: ranch	5
Salad: mixed greens	0
Salsa : fat-free	0

Food	Points
Shrimp: 3oz: cooked	1
Spinach	0
Strawberries	0
Sugar: 1 tsp: granulated: white	1
Sweet Potatoes: 1/2 cup: cooked	3
Sweet red peppers	0
Tomatoes	0
Tortilla chips : 1oz	4
Tortilla (flour) : 1 oz. or 1 medium	3
Tuna fish: 3oz: canned in water	1
Turkey bacon: 3 slices: cooked	3
Water	0
Watermelon	0
White rice: 1 cup: cooked	6
White wine: 5oz	4
Yogurt: 1 cup: Greek: fat-free: plain	3
Zucchini	0

Take Time to Indulge: Your Weekly 35 Flexible Points

The Weight Watchers diet program allows you to use 35 flexible Smart Points per week – consider it as your fun points. You have an option to use them or leave them. Remember, you cannot carry over the unused flexible points to the succeeding week.

Here are the things that you can do with your flexible points on top of your daily Smart Points allowance:

1. Spread the flexible points evenly.

If you have 30 Smart Points to spend daily, you can add 7 points for a total of 37 daily Smart Points allowance. You can adjust the distribution as you see fit. If you have more workload in the afternoon, then adjust the points that you need to consume for lunch. You can also choose to adjust your snacks.

2. You can use it all at once.

If you and your friends have decided to meet over the weekend, then you can use your flexible points in one go. You won't feel awkward and guilty. You can also use it during special occasions such as family reunion, weddings, or company events.

3. Don't use it at all.

If you think that you are fine with your current Smart Points allowance, then don't bother using your flexible points at all.

Now you're ready to make a plan, but take a look at some of the scrumptious recipes.

The Smart Points of the recipes in this chapter as well as the succeeding chapters have been properly calculated to give you a worry-free meal planning. Keep in mind that the indicated Smart Points value is good only for one serving size.

Here are some of the recipes that can help you feel great in the morning.

Breakfast Recipes

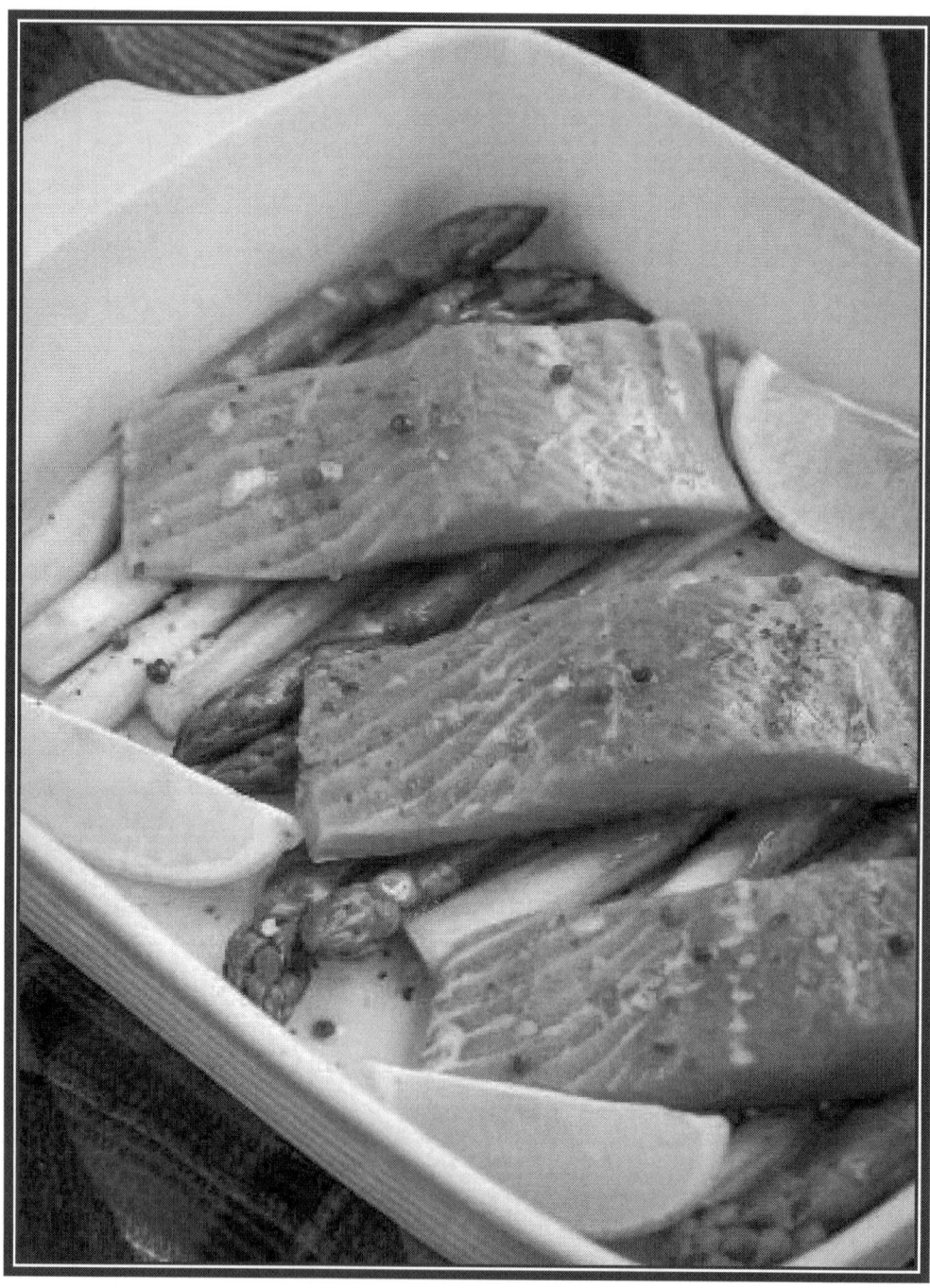

Mediterranean Strata with Goat Cheese

Prep Time	:	18 minutes
Cook Time	:	82 minutes
Smart Points per serving	:	6
1 Serving	:	1 slice

This recipe is good for 6 servings.

You will need:

- 1 tbsp. unsalted butter
- 1 large red onion, chopped
- 8oz cremini mushrooms, thinly sliced
- 3 cups regular liquid egg substitute
- 2oz semi-soft goat cheese, crumbled
- 1 tsp salt-free Italian seasoning
- 1/2 cup red peppers, roasted and coarsely chopped
- 1/2 cup sun-dried tomatoes in oil, coarsely chopped
- 10 slices reduced-calorie wheat bread (crust removed), cubed
- 1 tsp kosher salt
- 1/8 tsp black pepper
- Cooking spray

How to do it:

Preheat oven to 350°F.

Put a large skillet over medium heat and add butter. Add the onion and mushrooms. Add salt and pepper. Stir frequently until the mushrooms begin to brown. Stir in peppers and remove the pan from heat. Add Italian seasoning and tomatoes in the pan. Add the cubed bread and toss gently.

Get the cooking spray and coat oil all over the casserole dish. Pour the vegetable-bread mixture. Sprinkle the cheese and pour the egg substitute on top. Bake for 1 hour. Slice into 6 pieces and serve.

Cheesy and Saucy Egg Sandwich

Prep Time	:	13 minutes
Cook Time	:	11 minutes
Smart Points per serving	:	8
1 Serving	:	1 sandwich

This recipe is good for 2 servings.

You will need:

4 slices reduced-calorie rye bread, toasted

Things you will need for the Cheese Sauce:

- 1/4 cup low-fat cheddar cheese (sharp), shredded
- 1/4 cup skim milk, zero fat
- Dash of hot pepper sauce
- 3 tbsps. fat-free evaporated milk
- 2 tsp all-purpose flour
- Pinch of black pepper
- Pinch of salt

Things you will need for the Scrambled Eggs:

- 3 large egg whites
- 2 whole eggs
- 1 tbsp. skim milk, zero fat
- 1 tsp canola oil
- Pinch of black pepper
- Pinch of salt

How to do the Cheese Sauce:

Put a saucepan over medium heat. Mix flour, evaporated milk, and skim milk in a bowl. Add salt, pepper, and hot pepper sauce. Pour the mixture into the saucepan. Stir constantly until the mixture becomes thick. Reduce the heat and add cheese to the mixture. Continue to stir until smooth. Let it rest for a while.

How to do the Scrambled Eggs:

Get the ingredients for the scrambled eggs. Get a bowl and beat all the ingredients, except canola oil.

Prepare a large pan and put it over medium heat. Add the oil and heat it for a while. Add the egg mixture and scramble for at least 2 minutes.

How to assemble:

Get the toasted rye bread and put two on a flat surface. Divide the scrambled eggs equally among the two toasts. Add cheese sauce and top with the remaining toasts. Serve.

Hash and Eggs

Prep Time	:	15 minutes
Cook Time	:	51 minutes
Smart Points per serving	:	8
1 Serving	:	1 egg + 3/4 cup hash

This recipe is good for 4 servings.

You will need:

- 1/3 pound turkey pastrami, coarsely chopped
- 4 medium potatoes, cut into bite-size pieces
- 1/2 cup fresh cherry tomatoes
- 1/2 tsp rosemary, finely chopped
- 4 large eggs
- 1 tbsp. olive oil
- 1 1/2 cups onion, thinly sliced
- 1 1/2 cups red peppers, roasted and thinly sliced
- 1 tsp salt
- 1 tsp black pepper
- Cooking sprays

How to do it:

Preheat oven to 450°F. Prepare a 9-inch x 13-inch oven-proof pan and coat it with cooking spray.

Boil water in a medium pan. Add potatoes and parboil them for about 5 to 6 minutes.

Combine potatoes, pastrami, roasted peppers, onions, tomatoes, salt, black pepper, and rosemary in the prepared pan. Add oil and toss. Bake for about 30 to 45 minutes. Rotate the dish once or twice while cooking.

Get another skillet and fry the eggs. Serve.

Creamy Scrambled Eggs with Scallions and Tomatoes

Prep Time	:	8 minutes
Cook Time	:	3 minutes
Smart Points per serving	:	4
1 Serving	:	3/4 cup

This recipe is good for 4 servings.

You will need:

- 4 large whole eggs
- 4 large egg whites
- 1/3 cup scallions, sliced
- 3/4 cup fresh tomatoes, diced
- 2oz low-fat cream cheese, cut into bits
- 1/2 tsp salt
- 1/8 tsp black pepper
- Cooking spray

How to do it:

Get a medium skillet and coat it with cooking spray. Put it over medium heat.

Whisk eggs, salt, scallions, egg whites, and pepper in a medium bowl. Blend well. Pour the egg mixture into the skillet. Cook for about two minutes. Make sure to gently turn the mixture using a wooden spoon.

Add in cheese and tomatoes. Cook for 1 minute over low heat while stirring.

Steak and Eggs

Prep Time	:	7 minutes
Cook Time	:	8 minutes
Smart Points per serving	:	5
1 Serving	:	2oz beef + 1/4 omelette + sauce

This recipe is good for 4 servings.

You will need:

- 8oz deli style roast beef, thickly sliced
- 2 tbsps. club soda
- 4 large whole eggs
- 3 tbsps. steak sauce
- 4 large egg whites
- Salt and black pepper to taste
- Cooking spray

How to do it:

Get a large nonstick skillet and coat it with cooking spray. Put it over medium heat.

Whisk eggs, club soda, and egg whites in a bowl until frothy. Pour the mixture into the pan. Cook until underside becomes firm. Flip eggs over. Cook the other side for about 2 to 3 minutes. Transfer the omelet to a plate and keep it warm.

Put the roast beef to the skillet. Cook for about 1 to 2 minutes, and don't forget to flip once.

Cut the omelet into four equal parts and season with salt and pepper.

Serve each one with 2 ounces roast beef, 2 1/4 teaspoons steak sauce, and a quarter of omelet.

Passion Fruit Soufflé Omelette and Blueberries

Prep Time	:	10 minutes
Cook Time	:	20 minutes
Smart Points per serving	:	4
1 Serving	:	1 omelette

This recipe is good for 4 servings.

You will need:

- 2 tbsps. caster sugar
- 125g fresh blueberries, divide into 4 portions
- 1 tbsp. flour
- 3 medium eggs, separate the yolks from the whites
- 1/4 cup fresh passion fruit pulp
- 1 medium fresh passion fruit, get the pulp
- 1 tsp icing sugar
- Cooking spray

How to do it:

Preheat oven to 350°F. Beat the egg yolks, caster sugar, and 1/4 cup passion fruit pulp in a large bowl. Get an electric mixer and beat the egg whites until foamy. Fold the egg whites into the egg yolk mixture and blend gently. Add flour to the mixture. Stir gently to combine the flour and the mixture.

Coat a 20cm ovenproof frying pan with some oil and put it over medium heat. Ladle a quarter of the mixture in the pan and scatter to coat the bottom of the pan. Cook for a minute and set aside. Repeat the same process with the rest of the mixture.

Arrange the 4 omelets in a baking dish and bake for 4 minutes. Remove from the oven and scatter 1/4 of the blueberries on half of the omelet. Fold the omelet and put it on a plate. Repeat the process until there's no more omelet.

Drizzle passion fruit pulp on each omelet and dust with icing sugar.

Mexican Breakfast Burritos

Prep Time	:	15 minutes
Cook Time	:	34 minutes
Smart Points per serving	:	4
1 Serving	:	1 burrito

This recipe is good for 6 servings.

You will need:

- 1 medium poblano chili, chopped
- 6 tbsps. fat-free salsa
- 1/2 medium onion, chopped
- 6 medium whole wheat tortillas
- 1 pinch cayenne pepper
- 3/4 cup reduced-fat Mexican blend cheese, shredded
- 2 cups regular liquid egg substitute
- 6 tbsps. reduced-fat sour cream
- 1 tsp ground cumin
- 3/4 tsp kosher salt
- Cooking spray

How to do it:

Preheat oven to 350°F.

Combine salsa and sour cream in a small bowl. Set aside.

Get the cooking spray and coat the large nonstick skillet. Put it over medium-high heat. Sauté onion and pepper for about 5 to 7 minutes.

Whisk the egg substitute, cayenne, cumin, and salt in a bowl. Pour the mixture into the skillet. Scramble mixture for about 10 to 12 minutes.

Put tortilla on a flat surface. Put 1/2 cup egg mixture in the center of tortilla. Add 2 tablespoons each of cheese and salsa mixture. Roll or fold the burrito and wrap with foil. Do the same with the rest of the burritos.

Arrange the burritos on a baking sheet and bake for 10 to 15 minutes. Serve.

Egg, Canadian Bacon, Avocado, and Tomato Sandwich

Prep Time	:	10 minutes
Cook Time	:	4 minutes
Smart Points per serving	:	6
1 Serving	:	1 sandwich

This recipe is good for 4 servings.

You will need:

- 4 pieces English muffin, split in two and toasted
- 4 slices Canadian bacon
- 3 large eggs
- 4 large egg whites
- 2 tbsps. scallion, sliced
- 1 medium tomato, cut into 8 slices
- Half of medium avocado, cut into 8 slices
- 1/2 tbsp. salt
- 1/4 tsp black pepper
- Cooking sprays

How to do it:

Get a large nonstick skillet and coat it with cooking spray. Put it over medium heat. Add bacon and cook for about 1 to 2 minutes. Make sure to turn the bacon slices once.

Transfer the cooked bacon to a plate. Put 1 bacon slice at the bottom half of each English muffin.

Use the same skillet and coat it with cooking spray once more. Put it over medium heat.

Beat egg whites, scallions, eggs, salt, and pepper in a bowl until blended. Pour the mixture into the skillet and scramble for 1 minute.

Put 1/4 of the scrambled eggs on each bacon. Add 2 tomato slices and 2 avocado slices on top. Cover with the English muffin top and serve.

Mini Zucchini Quiche

Prep Time	:	25 minutes
Cook Time	:	15 minutes
Smart Points per serving	:	1
1 Serving	:	1 quiche

This recipe is good for 48 servings.

You will need:

- 2 small zucchinis, finely chopped
- 1 cup parmesan cheese, shredded
- 1 tsp sugar
- 1 large onion, finely chopped
- 1/2 cup all-purpose flour, sifted
- 6 large eggs
- 3 tbsps. extra virgin olive oil
- 1/4 cup fresh basil, finely chopped
- 2 tsp baking powder
- 1 tsp kosher salt
- 1/2 tsp black pepper
- Cooking spray

How to do it:

Preheat oven to 375°F.

Prepare two mini muffin pans with 24 holes each. Coat each muffin hole with cooking spray.

Get a large bowl and combine all the ingredients. Put 1 tablespoonful egg mixture into each muffin hole.

Bake for about 15 minutes and check if cooked through. Remove the quiche from the oven. Cool before serving.

Italian Pepper and Egg Sandwich

Prep Time	:	10 minutes
Cook Time	:	12 minutes
Smart Points per serving	:	6
1 Serving	:	1 sandwich

This recipe is good for 4 servings.

You will need:

- 4 large whole eggs
- 3 large egg whites
- 1 tsp garlic, minced
- 1 small onions, thinly sliced
- 2 tsp olive oil
- 1 large green pepper, thinly sliced
- 1/2 tsp salt
- 1/4 tsp black pepper
- 4 pieces reduced-calorie hamburger rolls, lightly toasted

How to do it:

Put oil in a large nonstick skillet over medium heat. Sauté onion and pepper for about 7 minutes. Add garlic and cook for about 30 seconds. Set aside.

Beat egg whites, eggs, salt, and pepper together in a bowl. Pour the egg mixture into the skillet with onion and scramble over medium heat for 1 to 2 minutes.

Split each hamburger roll across and put 3/4 cup egg mixture on top of the bottom half of the roll. Cover each roll with their top part. Serve.

Fluffy Lemon-Ricotta Pancakes

Prep Time	:	10 minutes
Cook Time	:	18 minutes
Smart Points per serving	:	6
1 Serving	:	2 pancakes

This recipe is good for 6 servings.

You will need:

- 2 large eggs, separate the yolks and whites
- 1 cup low-fat buttermilk
- 1 tsp baking soda
- 2 tbsps. lemon zest
- 2 tbsps. granulated sugar
- 1 1/2 cups all-purpose flour
- 1/2 cup part-skim ricotta cheese
- 1/2 tsp table salt
- Cooking spray

How to do it:

Whisk baking soda, flour, and salt in a bowl. Set aside.

Beat the egg whites using an electric mixer until soft, firm peaks appear.

Get a large bowl and combine ricotta cheese, sugar, egg yolks, and buttermilk. Add the flour mixture to the ricotta cheese mixture. Fold in the egg whites to combine.

Prepare a large pan and coat it with cooking spray. Put it over medium heat. Pour 1/4 of batter to make 1 pancake. Cook each side for 2 to3 minutes. Do the same with the rest of the batter. Keep the pancakes warm.

Quinoa and Apple Breakfast Cereal

Prep Time	:	10 minutes
Cook Time	:	25 minutes
Smart Points per serving	:	6
1 Serving	:	2/3 cup

This recipe is good for 6 servings.

You will need:

- 2 medium fresh apples, coarsely chopped
- 3 tbsps. packed brown sugar
- 1 cup quinoa
- 1 tbsp. salted butter
- 2 cups cold water
- 1/2 cup fat-free skim milk
- 1/2 tsp ground cinnamon
- Cooking spray

How to do it:

Get a bowl and pour in some water. Soak quinoa in the bowl for 5 minutes.

Prepare a large skillet and coat it with cooking spray. Put it over medium heat. Add 1/2 tablespoon butter to melt and when it started sizzling, add the apples. Cook for about 5 to 10 minutes while flipping occasionally. Set aside.

Rinse and drain the quinoa first before transferring in a medium saucepan. Add 2 cups of water and bring to a boil. Reduce the heat, cover the pan, and let your quinoa simmer for 10 minutes.

The quinoa is cooked when a little "tail" appears on the grain. Remove from heat and use a fork to fluff the quinoa. Add sugar, cinnamon, milk, and the remaining butter. Mix well and fold in apples. Serve.

Whole-Grain Banana Pancakes with Blackberry Syrup

Prep Time	:	15 minutes
Cook Time	:	15 minutes
Smart Points per serving	:	6
1 Serving	:	2 pancakes + 2 tbsps. syrup

This recipe is good for 6 servings.

You will need:

- 2 medium bananas, thinly sliced
- 1/4 cup wheat germ
- 1/4 cup flaxseeds
- 1 tsp vanilla extract
- 2 cups fresh blackberries
- 1 cup fat-free skim milk
- 2 tbsps. powdered sugar
- 1 tbsp. walnut oil
- 1 cup pancake mix
- 3 large egg whites
- Cooking spray

How to do it:

Get a large nonstick skillet and coat it with cooking spray. Put it over medium fire and preheat.

Combine powdered sugar and blackberries in a saucepan. Put it over medium heat and wait for it to simmer. Cook the sauce until it thickens.

Get a large bowl and combine wheat germs, flaxseeds, and pancake mix. Add egg whites, vanilla extract, milk, and oil. Whisk until there are no more large lumps.

Pour 1/4 cup of batter into the preheated skillet. When the bubbles appear, put banana slices on the pancake. Flip the pancake and cook for 1 minute. Do the same to the rest of the mixture.

Transfer the cooked pancakes to a serving platter and make sure to keep them warm.

Cheesy Vegetable Sandwich

Prep Time	:	5 minutes
Cook Time	:	5 minutes
Smart Points per serving	:	6
1 Serving	:	1 sandwich

This recipe is good for 1 serving.

You will need:

- 1 bun of 100-calorie flat sandwich
- 1 slice 2% milk Swiss cheese
- 1/2 cup fat-free liquid egg substitute
- 1/2 cup spinach leaves, chopped
- 1 tbsp. finely chopped red onion

How to do it:

Get a microwave-safe bowl that is big enough to accommodate the sandwich bun. Coat the bowl with nonstick spray. Put the onion and spinach in the bowl and microwave until spinach wilts. Use a paper towel to absorb the excess moisture.

Stir in the egg substitute to the bowl of spinach and microwave for 1 minute. Stir it for one more time and microwave for another minute.

Get a microwave-safe plate and put the bottom half of the bun on it. Scoop the egg patty from the bowl and put it on the bun. Add cheese on top and cover it with the top half of the bun.

Microwave the sandwich for about 20 seconds.

French Toast Nuggets

Prep Time	:	5 minutes
Cook Time	:	5 minutes
Smart Points per serving	:	6
1 Serving	:	8 nuggets

This recipe is good for 1 serving.

You will need:

- 1 hot dog bun (standard size)
- Dash of cinnamon
- 1/4 tsp vanilla extract
- 2 tsp light butter, whipped
- 1/4 cup egg whites

How to do it:

Mix vanilla extract, egg whites, and cinnamon in a bowl that can accommodate the hot dog bun.

Slice the bun in two, lengthwise. Slice each half into 4 equal pieces, widthwise. You need to come up with 8 nuggets.

Dip each nugget in the egg mixture. Make sure to coat all sides of each nugget.

Prepare a skillet and spray it with nonstick spray. Put it over medium heat. Add butter and allow it to coat the surface of the skillet.

Cook the nuggets until all sides turn golden brown.

Oat and Apricot Bars

Prep Time	:	12 minutes
Cook Time	:	20 minutes
Smart Points per serving	:	7
1 Serving	:	1 bar

This recipe is good for 8 servings.

You will need:

- Half cup packed brown sugar
- 1 tbsp. reduced-calorie margarine, melted
- 15 pieces dried apricot halves, diced
- 1 cup whole-grain wheat flour
- 1/2 cup liquid egg substitute
- 1 tsp baking powder
- 1/2 cup quick oats
- 2 tbsps. sunflower seeds
- Cooking spray

How to do it:

Preheat oven to 350ºF. Prepare an 8-inch square baking dish and spray it with some oil.

Combine flour, sugar, baking powder, apricots, oats, and sunflower seeds in a bowl.

In another bowl, whisk the egg substitute and margarine. Combine the dry and wet ingredients and mix well. Transfer the mixture into the baking dish, and bake for about 20 minutes. Let it cool and cut it into 8 rectangles.

Bacon, Egg, and Spinach Stacks

Prep Time	:	15 minutes
Cook Time	:	55 minutes
Smart Points per serving	:	4
1 Serving	:	1 stack

This recipe is good for 12 servings.

You will need:

- 6 slices Canadian bacon, quartered
- 1 cup part-skim ricotta cheese
- 12oz bliss potatoes (baby-variety), steamed
- 2 large eggs, beaten
- 1 cup low-fat cheddar cheese, shredded
- 9oz fresh spinach (baby-variety), steamed and drained
- 2 tbsps. fresh chives, chopped

How to do it:

Preheat oven to 350°F.

Slice the steamed potato into 4 rounds. Set aside.

Get a bowl. Combine eggs, ricotta cheese, and chives.

Prepare a muffin pan and put a potato slice with a flat surface in each muffin hole. Top each potato slice with a quarter slice of bacon, 1 teaspoon of ricotta cheese mixture, 2 tablespoons steamed spinach, 1 tablespoon cheddar cheese, and another quarter slice of bacon. Top it with 1 teaspoon of ricotta mixture on top of each muffin hole. Place the remaining slices of potato on top and sprinkle with the remaining cheese.

Bake for about 30 to 35 minutes. Let it cool for about 10 to 15 minutes before transferring the stacks to the rack. Serve.

Chicken BLT Sandwich

Prep Time	:	10 minutes
Cook Time	:	n/a
Smart Points per serving	:	7
1 Serving	:	1 sandwich

This recipe is good for 1 serving.

You will need:

- 3oz skinless chicken breast, pre-cooked and finely chopped
- 1/2 tsp lemon juice
- 1 tbsp. chopped scallions
- 2 medium lettuce leaves
- 2 slices light wheat bread
- 1 tbsp. crumbled bacon, pre-cooked
- 1 tbsp. sun-dried tomatoes, finely chopped
- 1 tbsp. light mayonnaise
- Dash black pepper

How to do it:

Combine lemon juice, mayonnaise, and pepper in a bowl. Stir well. Add the remaining ingredients, except lettuce. Blend well to distribute the flavors evenly.

Put a lettuce leaf on top of a slice of bread, followed by the chicken mixture. Top it with another lettuce leaf and cover with the remaining bread slice.

Denver Omelette in a Mug

Prep Time	:	5 minutes
Cook Time	:	5 minutes
Smart Points per serving	:	2
1 Serving	:	1 mug

This recipe is good for 1 serving.

You will need:

- 2 slices fat-free ham, chopped
- 2 tbsps. onion, chopped
- 1/4 cup green bell pepper, chopped
- 2 tbsps. fat-free cheddar cheese, shredded
- 1/2 cup fat-free liquid egg substitute

How to do it:

Prepare a large microwave-safe mug and coat it with nonstick spray. Add the onion and pepper, and microwave for 1 1/2 minutes.

Use a paper towel to absorb the excess moisture. Stir in egg substitute and microwave for another minute.

Add ham and cheese, and microwave for 1 minute or until set.

Pork Recipes

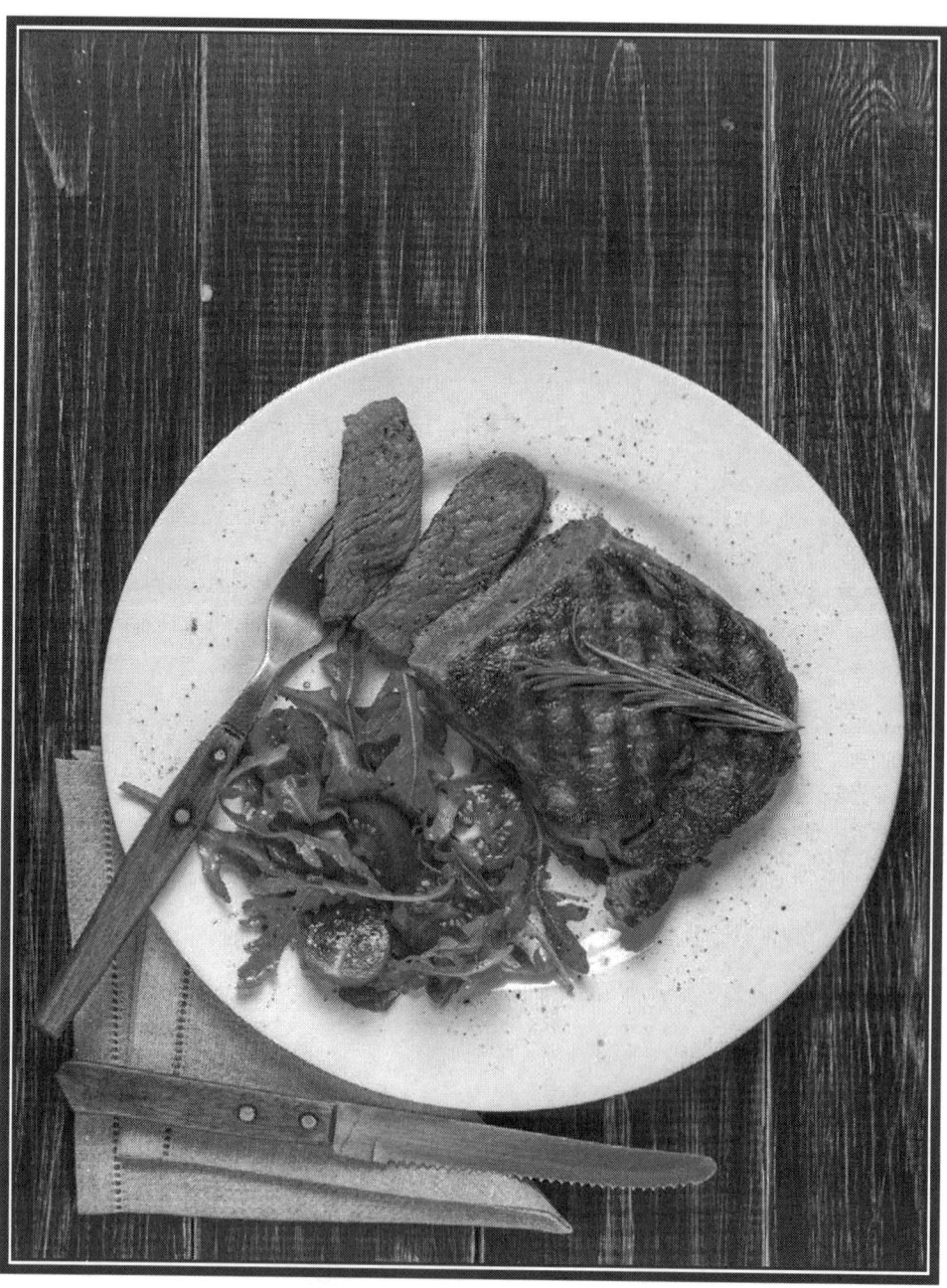

These pork recipes are simply succulent and delicious. You and your family will surely enjoy eating them time and again.

Spice-Rubbed Pork Chops

Prep Time	:	10 minutes
Cook Time	:	8 minutes
Smart Points per serving	:	5
1 Serving	:	1 pork chop + string beans

This recipe is good for 4 servings.

You will need:

- 4 pieces lean pork chops that weigh 0.5 pounds each
- 1tsp garlic powder
- 1/2 tsp lemon juice, freshly squeezed
- 1 tbsp. brown sugar
- 1 1/2 tbsps. chili powder
- 2 tsp cumin, ground
- 2 tbsps. Worcestershire sauce
- 1 pound green snap beans, steamed
- String beans for garnishing

How to do it:

Preheat the broiler. Cover the pan with cooking spray.

Combine garlic powder, sugar, cumin, and chili powder in a bowl. Add Worcestershire sauce. Mix everything into a paste, and divide it into 4 equal parts.

Use one part of the mixture for each pork chop. Make sure to rub the mixture on both sides of the pork chops.

Arrange the chops on the pan and broil 4 minutes. Flip the chops and broil the other side until cooked

Splash the lemon juice on the string beans. Serve.

Pork Tenderloin Roast

Prep Time	:	15 minutes
Cook Time	:	36 minutes
Smart Points per serving	:	3
1 Serving	:	3 ounces tenderloin

This recipe is good for 6 servings.

Ingredients:

- 2 pounds lean pork tenderloin
- 1 tsp garlic powder
- 2 tsp thyme, dried
- 1 tsp onion powder
- 2 tsp olive oil
- 2 tsp oregano, dried
- 1 tsp black pepper, ground
- 1 tsp table salt
- Cooking spray

How to do it:

Set the oven to 400ºF. Get a roasting pan and coat it with oil.

Mix garlic powder, oregano, thyme, salt, pepper, and onion powder in a bowl. Set aside.

Massage olive oil to the tenderloin and roll it in the mixture. Coat the tenderloin well. Put it in the pan.

Roast the meat for about 25 to 30 minutes. Insert a meat thermometer in the center of the tenderloin. If the temperature is 145ºF, you can take it out of the pan.

Let the cooked pork rest for 3 minutes. Slice and serve.

Seasoned Pork Tenderloin

Prep Time	:	10 minutes
Cook Time	:	10 minutes
Smart Points per serving	:	4
1 Serving	:	1 slice of tenderloin

This recipe is good for 8 servings.

You will need:

- 2 pieces of 1 1/4 pound lean pork tenderloin
- 1/2 cup reduced-calorie pancake syrup
- 1 tsp ginger, ground
- 1 tsp cloves, ground
- 1/2 tsp cinnamon, ground
- 1 tsp dry mustard
- Salt and pepper to taste

How to do it:

Combine syrup, dry mustard, ginger, cloves, salt, cinnamon, and pepper in a bowl. Put the mixture inside a large resealable plastic bag.

Remove the pork fat. You need to come up with 8 tenderloin slices. Put the tenderloin slices in the plastic bag with the syrup mixture. Shake the bag to coat each piece of meat with the ginger mixture.

Put the plastic bag on a plate. Refrigerate the tenderloin in a bag. Turn the content occasionally. Let it marinade in the refrigerator for at least 2 hours. You can also let it sit overnight.

Preheat the broiler. Put the meat in a roasting dish. Brush the marinade over the meat pieces as you roast. Don't let the meat pieces directly touch the heat. If the temperature of the meat center reads 145°F, the tenderloin pieces are cooked.

Roast Pork Dinner

Prep Time	:	15 minutes
Cook Time	:	15 minutes
Smart Points per serving	:	7
1 Serving	:	3oz pork + 1/2 cup veggies + 1/2 cup potatoes

This recipe is good for 8 servings.

You will need:

- 2 pounds lean pork loin (it should be a whole piece of meat)
- 1 1/4 pounds red-variety baby potatoes, cut the large ones in half
- 2 tbsps. olive oil, extra-virgin
- 4 cloves garlic, minced
- 1 large red onion, cut into 12 wedges
- 2 medium green peppers, cut each pepper into 8 slices
- 1 1/2 tsp dried oregano
- 1 tbsp. fennel seed
- 1 1/2 tsp salt
- 1 1/4 tsp black pepper
- Cooking spray

How to do it:

Preheat oven to 400ºF.

Line a large roasting pan with aluminum foil and spray some cooking oil on it.

In a small bowl, mix fennel seeds, 1 tablespoon oil, garlic, oregano, 1 teaspoon pepper, and 1 teaspoon salt. Coat the pork with the mixture and put it in the roasting pan together with the potatoes and other vegetables.

Drizzle remaining oil over the vegetables and pork. Sprinkle the rest of the salt and pepper.

Leave the pan uncovered and roast for about 45 to 55 minutes. Turn the vegetables and potatoes once in a while. When the inserted meat thermometer reads 145ºF, the pork is done. Check the vegetables if they are tender enough.

Take the roasting pan out of the oven and rest it on a rack for 5 minutes. Slice the pork and serve it together with the potatoes and vegetables.

Cider-Glazed Pork Chops with Apples and Cabbage

Prep Time	:	18 minutes
Cook Time	:	32 minutes
Smart Points per serving	:	9
Serving	:	1 pork chop + 1/4 cabbage mixture

This recipe is good for 4 servings.

You will need:

- 1 1/4 pounds boneless pork chops (make it 4 pieces chops with the same weight)
- 2 tsp caraway seeds
- 2 large red onions, thinly sliced
- 2 large apples, peeled and diced
- 3 cups apple cider
- 3 1/2 cups red cabbage, shredded
- 1 tbsp. Dijon Mustard
- 1 cup reduced-sodium chicken broth
- 2 tsp olive oil, extra virgin
- 2 1/2 tsp salt
- 1/2 tsp black pepper, ground

How to do it:

Mix cider, broth, mustard, 1 teaspoon salt, and caraway seeds in a large bowl.

Put a large skillet over high heat. Add salt and pepper to the pork. When the skillet is hot enough, add some oil. Drop the pork into the skillet and cook each side until it turns golden brown. Transfer the cooked pork to the plate.

Sauté the onions in the same skillet and add salt. Stir constantly until the onions caramelized.

Add the apples in the skillet. Add the pork chops. Pour the cider mixture, cover the skillet, and bring it to a boil. Remove the cover and cook the chops for 5 minutes.

Add cabbage and stir occasionally. Cook for about 2 minutes.

Transfer the pork chops to a cutting board and let them cool for a bit.

Use a slotted spoon when transferring the cabbage mixture to a large serving bowl.

Boil the cider mixture until it thickens a bit. Divide the cabbage mixture into four portions. Serve the pork with cabbage mixture and glaze.

Pulled Pork Special

Prep Time	:	16 minutes
Cook Time	:	240 minutes
Smart Points per serving	:	6
1 Serving	:	1/6 of the recipe

This recipe is good for 6 servings.

You will need:

- 12oz boneless pork shoulder, trim excess fat
- 12oz lean boneless pork tenderloin, trim excess fat
- 2 tbsps. plus 2 tsp unpacked brown sugar
- 2 tbsps. plus 2 tsp cider vinegar
- 1/2 cup ketchup
- 2 tsp garlic powder
- 2 cups roughly chopped onion
- 1 cup canned tomato sauce
- 1/4 tsp salt
- 1/8 tsp black pepper

How to do it:

Combine ketchup, tomato sauce, garlic powder, sugar, and vinegar in a slow cooker. Season the pork shoulder and tenderloin with salt and pepper. Put the meat in the pot. Add onion and stir gently.

Close the slow cooker and cook on high for 3 to 4 hours.

Place the pork in a large bowl. Get two forks and use them to shred the meat. Put the shredded pork back in the slow cooker. Mix well and serve.

Sesame-Ginger Pork Tenderloin

Prep Time	:	10 minutes
Cook Time	:	35 minutes
Smart Points per serving	:	6
1 Serving	:	1/4 of the sliced pork + 1 cup veggies

This recipe is good for 4 servings.

You will need:

- 1/2 cup sesame ginger dressing
- 1 cup red onion, sliced
- 1 1/4 pounds pork tenderloin, cut off excess fat
- 6 cups kale, chopped
- 1 1/2 cups mushrooms, sliced
- Salt and black pepper

How to do it:

Put 1/4 cup dressing in a large bowl and add in pork. Gently massage the dressing into the pork and refrigerate for an hour.

Preheat oven to 425°F.

Get a large oven-safe skillet and coat it with nonstick spray. Put the skillet over medium heat. Add the meat in the skillet and sear each side evenly. Cook until all sides turn a bit brown.

Put the skillet in the oven. Bake for about 12 minutes. Take out the skillet and flip the pork. Return it to the oven and bake for another 8 or 10 minutes.

Transfer the cooked pork to a platter and cover loosely with foil for about 10 minutes.

Scrape off the bits from the skillet and coat it with another layer of cooking spray. Put it over medium-high heat. Add onions, mushrooms, a pinch of salt, and dash of pepper. Stir and cook for about 3 minutes.

Pour in half cup of water. Add kale. Stir, cover, and cook for another 3 minutes. Uncover and continue cooking for 2 to 3 minutes or until the liquid has significantly reduced.

Slice pork into bite-size pieces and serve with veggies.

Breaded Pork Cutlet

Prep Time	:	15 minutes
Cook Time	:	15 minutes
Smart Points per serving	:	7
1 Serving	:	1 pork cutlet + 1 lemon wedge

This recipe is good for 4 servings.

You will need:

- 4 pieces 4oz-pork chops, boneless
- 1/2 cup coarse breadcrumbs
- 1/2 cup flour
- 1 large egg
- 1/2 medium lemon, make 4 wedges
- 1 1/2 tsp Dijon mustard
- 3/4 tsp salt
- 1/2 tsp black pepper, ground
- 3 tbsps. skim milk, choose the fat-free variety
- Cooking spray

How to do it:

Preheat oven to 400°F. Prepare a baking pan and coat it with cooking spray.

Pound each pork chop until you get the 1/4-inch thickness. You can use a rolling pin to pound and smooth out the chops.

Mix salt, flour, and pepper in a bowl.

Beat the egg in another bowl. Add the mustard and milk in the beaten egg.

Spread the breadcrumbs on a plate.

Toss each chop in the flour mixture and coat well. Shake off the excess flour.

Dump each chop in the egg mixture and coat well.

Cover each side of the chop with breadcrumbs.

Coat your baking sheet with cooking spray.

Arrange the chops in the baking sheet and bake for 8 minutes. Flip each chop and continue baking for 5 to 7 minutes.

Serve each chop with a lemon wedge.

Spicy Asian Pork Tenderloin

Prep Time	:	15 minutes
Cook Time	:	30 minutes
Smart Points per serving	:	5
1 Serving	:	1/4 of recipe

This recipe is good for 4 servings.

You will need:

1 pound pork tenderloin, cut off excess fat

Things you will need for the marinade:

- 1 tsp red pepper flakes, crushed
- 2 tsp garlic, minced
- 2 tbsps. reduced-sodium soy sauce
- 1 tbsp. sweet Asian chili sauce
- 1 tsp ginger, chopped

Things you will need for the sauce:

- 3 tbsps. sweet Asian chili sauce
- 2 tbsps. thinly sliced scallions
- 2 tsp cornstarch
- 1/4 cup water
- 1/4 tsp red pepper flakes, crushed
- 1 tsp garlic, minced
- 1 1/2 tbsps. seasoned rice vinegar

How to do it:

Gather the ingredients for the marinade and dump them all in a bowl. Make sure to blend everything well. Put the pork in the marinade and gently massage the marinade into the meat. Cover and refrigerate for an hour.

Preheat oven to 425°F.

Prepare a large oven-safe skillet, coat it with cooking spray, and preheat it. Arrange the pork pieces in the skillet. Sear the meat evenly by flipping occasionally. Do it for about 4 minutes or until all sides are dark enough.

Pop the skillet in the oven. Bake for 10 minutes.

Flip the pork once and continue baking until the temperature in center reaches 145°F.

Take out the pork from the oven and transfer to a platter. Let it rest for 10 minutes.

To make the sauce, dissolve cornstarch in a small pot with water. Add the remaining ingredients for the sauce, except scallions. Mix well. Put the pot over medium heat while stirring frequently. Cook until the sauce thickens. Remove the pot from heat, and add the scallions.

Slice the pork and serve together with sauce.

Bacon-Bundled BBQ Shrimp

Prep Time	:	15 minutes
Cook Time	:	15 minutes
Smart Points per serving	:	4
1 Serving	:	4 shrimps

This recipe is good for 4 servings.

You will need:

- 16 pieces large shrimp (not jumbo), peeled and deveined
- 3 tbsps. ketchup
- 8 slices turkey bacon, cut in 2
- 1/3 cup canned tomato sauce
- 1/2 tsp garlic powder
- 1 tbsp. unpacked brown sugar
- 1 tbsp. apple cider vinegar

How to do it:

Preheat oven to 425°F. Coat the baking sheet with nonstick spray.

Get a medium bowl and combine tomato sauce, sugar, vinegar, garlic powder, and ketchup.

Dip each half-slice bacon in the sauce mixture, and wrap it around a shrimp. Secure with a wooden toothpick if needed. Put the bacon-wrapped shrimp on the baking sheet. Do the same with the rest of the shrimps.

Put the baking sheet in the oven and bake for 10 to 15 minutes or until shrimps are cooked through.

Beef Recipes

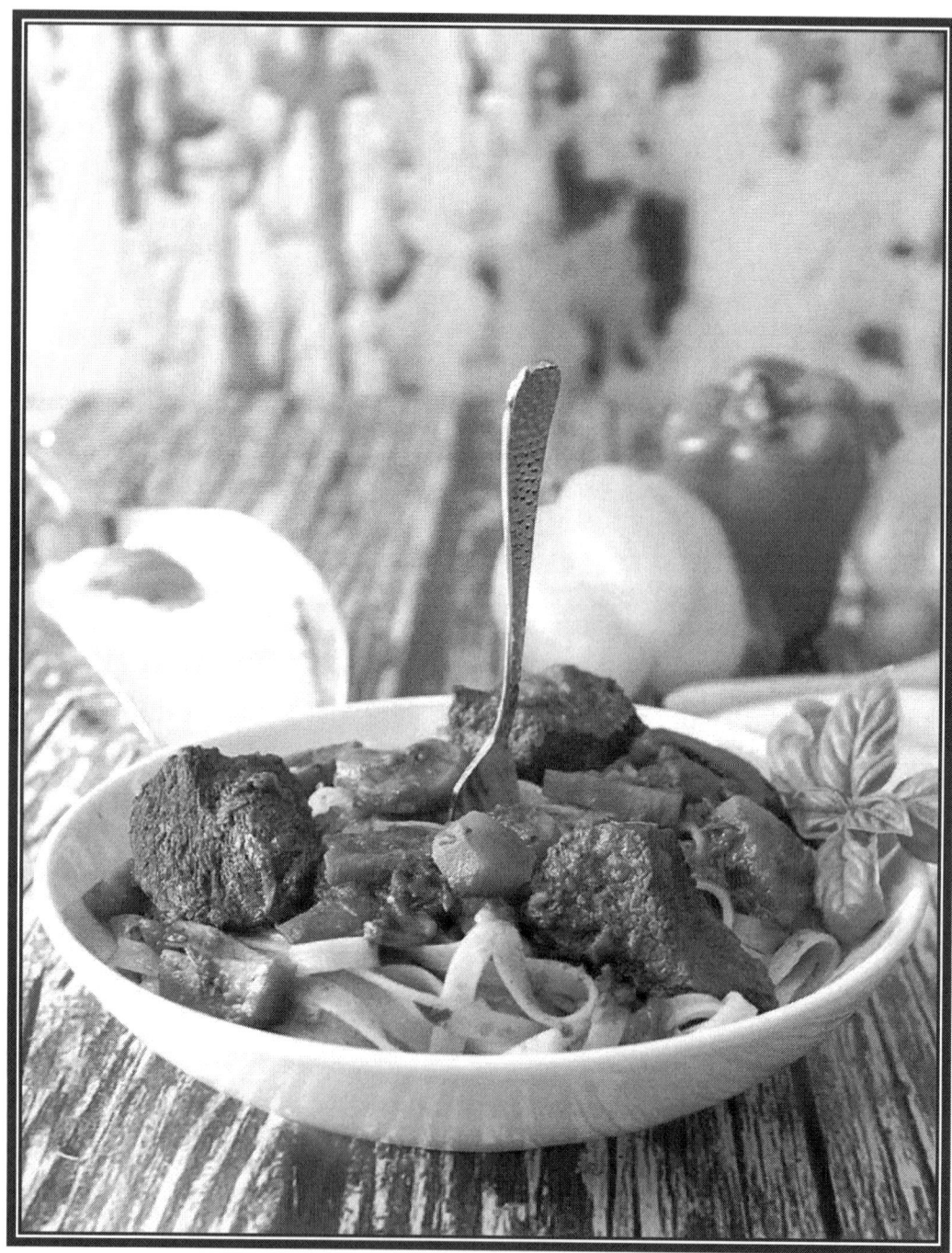

Try these beef recipes and be amazed.

Roasted Sirloin Beef

Prep Time	:	10 minutes
Cook Time	:	20 minutes
Smart Points per serving	:	2
1 Serving	:	3 ounces beef

This recipe is good for 8 servings.

You will need:

- 2 pounds lean sirloin beef, trimmed
- 2 tbsps. fresh rosemary, finely chopped
- 4 cloves garlic, minced
- 2 tbsps. fresh oregano, finely chopped
- 1 tsp salt
- 1/2 tsp black pepper, ground
- Cooking spray

How to do it:

Preheat oven to 400ºF.

Prepare a shallow pan for roasting. Spray oil to cover the surface.

Season the beef with salt and pepper. Place and arrange the meat in the pan.

Mix garlic, oregano, and rosemary in a bowl. Spread the herb mixture on top of the sirloin. Gently massage the mixture into the beef to bind it onto the sirloin.

Roast the meat for about 20 minutes or cooked. Let it sit on a rack for 5 minutes to cool.

Filet Mignon with Red Wine Sauce

Prep Time	:	10 minutes
Cook Time	:	18 minutes
Smart Points per serving	:	6
1 Serving	:	3 1/2 ounces steak + 1/2 of asparagus + 1 tbsp. sauce

This recipe is good for 2 servings.

You will need:

- 8oz lean beef filet mignon
- 1/2 pound asparagus, trimmed and steamed or roasted
- 6 tbsps. Burgundy or Bordeaux
- 1/2 tbsp. fresh chives or parsley, chopped
- 1 tsp unsalted butter
- 1/2 tsp each of salt and black pepper
- Cooking spray

How to do it:

Prepare a grill pan and coat it with cooking spray. Put it over medium-high heat.

Blend salt and pepper in a bowl. Rub the mixture all over the beef filet. When the pan is hot enough, add the beef filet and cook each side for about 4 minutes.

Arrange the cooked beef filet on a cutting board and cover with aluminum foil on top to keep it warm for at least 10 minutes.

Pour wine in a grill pan over high heat. You need to reduce the liquid by 75%. Scrape the bits that get stuck on the sides and bottom of the pan. Continue to simmer the sauce.

Add butter to the simmering sauce over low heat. Continue to stir until the butter melts.

Slice the beef. Put the slices on the plates. Add some sauce, garnish with chives or parsley, and serve with asparagus.

Buffalo Ranch Meatloaf

Prep Time	:	10 minutes
Cook Time	:	50 minutes
Smart Points per serving	:	3
1 Serving	:	1/5 of meatloaf

This recipe is good for 5 servings.

You will need:

- 1 1/4 pounds extra-lean ground beef
- 2 tbsps. cayenne pepper sauce
- 1/4 cup egg whites
- 2 tbsps. ranch dressing
- 1/4 tsp garlic powder
- 1/4 tsp black pepper

How to do it:

Preheat oven to 400ºF.

Coat the loaf pan with nonstick spray.

Get a large bowl, combine egg whites, beef, 1 tablespoon hot sauce, ranch mix, black pepper, and garlic powder. Mix well.

Pour the mixture into the loaf pan. Smooth out the surface. Put the pan in the oven and bake for about 50 minutes or until cooked through.

Top with the remaining hot sauce before slicing.

Bacon Cheeseburger Chili

Prep Time	:	15 minutes
Cook Time	:	240 minutes
Smart Points per serving	:	5
1 Serving	:	1 portion of chili + 1 tbsp. cheese + 1 tbsp. crumbled bacon

This recipe is good for 7 servings.

You will need:

- 7 tbsps. reduced-fat cheddar cheese, shredded
- 2 tsp yellow mustard
- 1 pound extra-lean ground beef
- 14.5oz-can diced tomatoes, do not drain
- 1 cup tomatoes, finely chopped
- 2 tbsps. Worcestershire sauce
- 1 cup bell pepper, chopped
- 4 slices bacon
- 2 tsp garlic, minced
- 1 cup onion, chopped
- 1/2 cup ketchup
- 15oz-can red kidney beans, rinsed and drained
- 1 tsp ground cumin
- 2 tsp chili powder

How to do it:

Coat a slow cooker with nonstick spray.

Combine finely chopped tomatoes, mustard, Worcestershire sauce, and ketchup in a large bowl. Mix until well blended. Add onion, diced tomatoes, beans, and pepper. Stir well.

Put the beef in a slow cooker. Add garlic, cumin, and chili powder. Combine well. Add the saucy veggie mixture and stir thoroughly to break up the meat.

Close the slow cooker and cook on high for 3 to 4 hours. The veggies must be softened and the beef must be thoroughly cooked. Stir well.

Put a nonstick skillet over medium heat and cook bacon until crispy.

Divide the beef and veggies into 7 equal portions. Top each portion with cheese and crumbled bacon.

100-Calorie Beef Patties

Prep Time	:	10 minutes
Cook Time	:	20 minutes
Smart Points per serving	:	2
1 Serving	:	1 beef patty

This recipe is good for 6 servings.

You will need:

- 1 pound extra-lean ground beef
- 1/4 tsp onion powder
- 1/4 tsp garlic powder
- 1/4 cup liquid egg whites
- 1/2 tsp salt
- 1/2 tsp black pepper

How to do it:

Dump all the ingredients in a large bowl. Mix well and make sure that everything is evenly distributed. Divide the mixture into 6 equal portions and form them into patties. Prepare a large skillet and coat it with cooking spray. Put it over medium heat.

Add the patties and cook each side for 4 minutes.

Stir-Fry Beef and Broccoli

Prep Time	:	16 minutes
Cook Time	:	12 minutes
Smart Points per serving	:	3
1 Serving	:	1 1/4 cups beef and broccoli

This recipe is good for 4 servings.

You will need:

- 3/4 pound lean sirloin beef, sliced into strips
- 4 cloves garlic, minced
- 5 cups broccoli, cut into florets
- 2 1/2 tbsps. cornstarch
- 2 tsp canola oil
- 1/4 cup low sodium soy sauce
- 1 tbsp. fresh ginger, grated
- 1/4 tsp red pepper flakes
- 1 cup reduced-sodium chicken broth
- 1/4 cup water
- 1/4 tsp salt

How to do it:

Sift cornstarch on a plate and add salt. Mix well. Coat the beef strips with the mixture.

Prepare a wok and put it over medium-high heat. Add some oil. Add the beef strips and stir-fry until lightly browned. Transfer the cooked beef to a bowl.

Use the same wok and add a half cup of broth. Scrape the bottom of the pan to loosen the stuck bits.

Stir in the broccoli florets. You may need to add more water to make the florets tender. Add garlic, red pepper flakes, and ginger. Stir-fry for 1 minute.

Combine the rest of cornstarch, water, half cup broth, and soy sauce. Blend well and stir into the pan. Reduce the heat. Continue stirring until the sauce thickens.

Add the beef and the juices to the wok. Mix well to coat the beef with the sauce.

Steak and Mushroom with Mashies

Prep Time	:	10 minutes
Cook Time	:	30 minutes
Smart Points per serving	:	9
1 Serving	:	1 Beef filet + 1/3 cup mushrooms + 3/4 cup mashies

This recipe is good for 2 servings.

Things you will need for Steak and the Mushroom Topping:

- 2 pieces 6oz-filet lean beefsteak
- 1 1/2 tsp light butter
- 2 cups brown mushrooms, sliced
- Dash of thyme, ground
- 2 tbsps. sherry cooking wine
- Pinch of black pepper, ground
- 1/4 tsp salt

Things you will need for the Mashies:

- 6oz potatoes, peeled and cubed
- 1 1/2 cups cauliflower, cut into florets
- 1 1/2 tsp light butter
- 2 tbsps. light sour cream
- 1/8 tsp each of salt and black pepper

How to do it:

Fill a large pot with water and put it over high heat. Bring it to a boil.

Drop the potatoes first and soften for a bit before dropping the cauliflower florets. Cook for 15 to 20 minutes.

Pound the filets to get even thickness and season with salt and pepper. Coat a large skillet with cooking spray and put it over medium heat. Add in the filets and cover. Cook each side of the steak for 4 minutes. Transfer the cooked filets in a plate.

Remove the burnt bits and re-spray the skillet. Put it over medium heat. Stir in mushrooms and remaining salt. Cook until lightly browned. Add thyme, sherry, and butter. Continue cooking and stirring until the butter begins melting and coating the mushrooms evenly. Ladle the mixture and pour on the steaks.

Drain the potato and cauliflower. Place them in a large bowl, mash them. Add the rest of the ingredients for mashies and mix well.

Amazing Cheeseburger Patty

Prep Time	:	5 minutes
Cook Time	:	20 minutes
Smart Points per serving	:	4
1 Serving	:	1 cheeseburger patty

This recipe is good for 1 serving.

You will need:

- 4oz extra-lean ground beef
- 1 wedge light creamy Swiss cheese
- 1/8 tsp garlic powder
- 1/8 tsp Worcestershire sauce
- 1/8 tsp onion powder
- Salt and black pepper to taste

How to do it:

Get a medium bowl and put all the ingredients, except cheese. Mix everything well.

Shape the mixture into a ball. Poke the top of the ball with your thumb and make a hollow indentation towards the center or core of the meatball.

Fill the cavity with cheese and cover everything with the meat and seal the cheese inside. Gently press the ball to form a thick patty.

Put a nonstick grill pan with oil over medium heat. Cook each side of the patty for 4 to 8 minutes. Serve.

Chicken Recipes

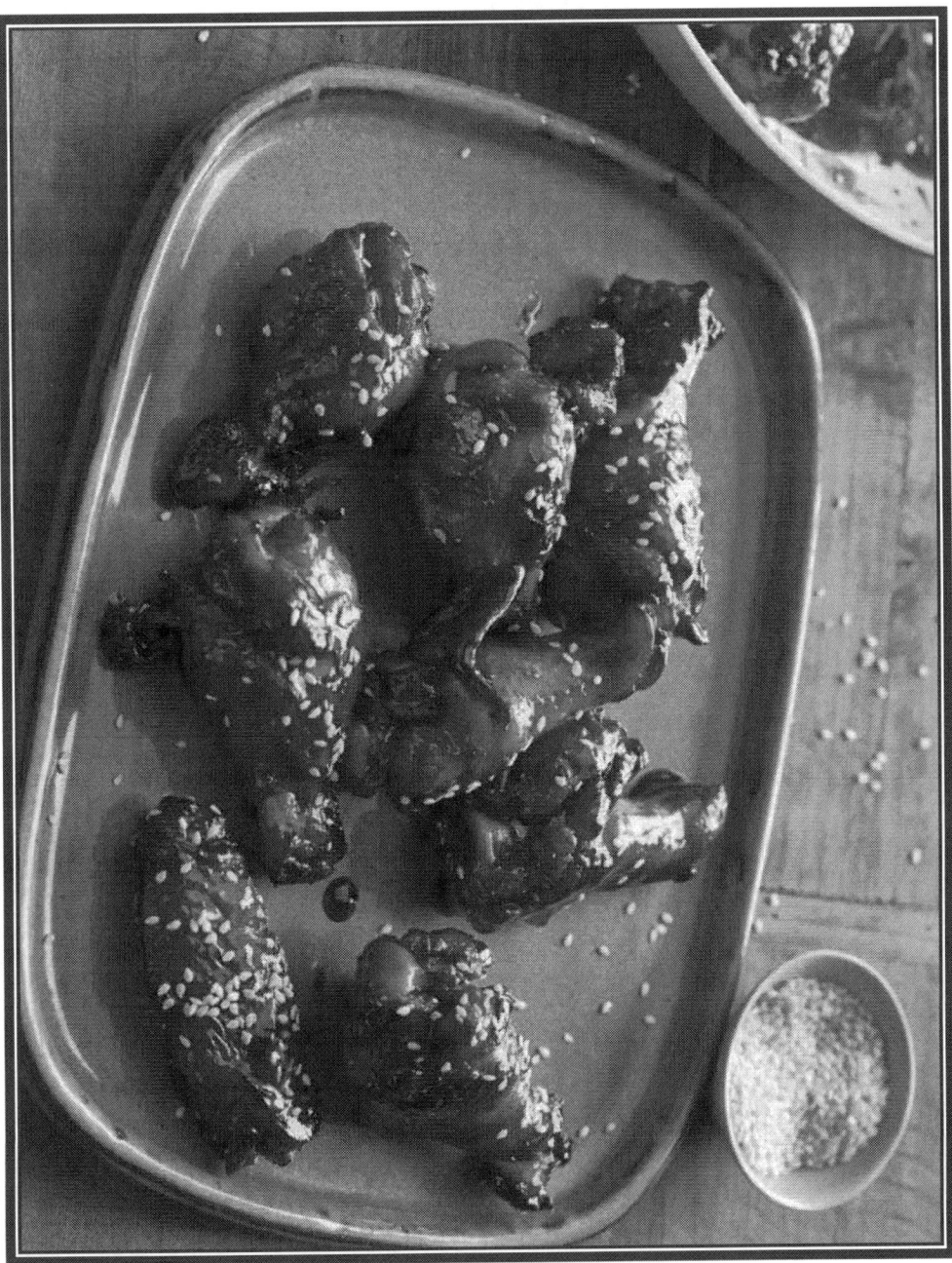

These chicken recipes are easy to do and simply delicious.

Baked Chicken

Prep Time	:	10 minutes
Cook Time	:	35 minutes
Smart Points per serving	:	2
1 Serving	:	1 chicken breast half

This recipe is good for 4 servings.

You will need:

- 1 pound chicken breast, boneless skinless
- 1/4 cup reduced-sodium chicken broth
- 1 tsp olive oil
- 2 tsp fresh parsley, chopped
- 2 tsp fresh lemon juice
- 2 tsp fresh rosemary, chopped
- 1/2 medium lemon, quartered
- 1/4 tsp black pepper, ground
- 1/2 tsp salt
- Cooking spray

How to do it:

Preheat oven to 400ºF.

Spray some oil on a shallow roasting pan.

Rub salt and pepper all over the chicken. Place the chicken in the roasting pan and splash some oil.

Combine lemon juice, parsley, and rosemary in a bowl. Coat the chicken with the lemon juice mixture. Add the broth to cover the bottom of the pan.

Put the chicken in the oven and bake for 30 to 35 minutes. Use the lemon wedges as garnishing.

Feta-Stuffed Chicken Burgers

Prep Time	:	15 minutes
Cook Time	:	16 minutes
Smart Points per serving	:	6
1 Serving	:	1 sandwich

This recipe is good for 4 servings.

You will need:

- 1 pound chicken breast, finely chopped
- 5 pieces black olive, pitted and sliced
- 4 pieces hamburger rolls (choose the reduced-calorie variety)
- 1/4 tsp garlic powder
- 1 tbsp. fresh oregano
- 7 tbsps. feta cheese, crumbled
- 1 cup romaine lettuce, coarsely chopped
- 2/3 cup red peppers, roasted and sliced

How to do it:

Preheat the grill.

Combine chicken, garlic powder, feta, and oregano in a bowl. Divide the mixture into four parts. Turn each part into a ball. Press each ball into a patty.

Grill each side of the patty for about 7 to 8 minutes.

To assemble: put a patty on the bottom half of the bun. Add olives, lettuce, and peppers. Cover it with the top of the bun to finish.

General Tso's Chicken

Prep Time	:	20 minutes
Cook Time	:	10 minutes
Smart Points per serving	:	8
1 Serving	:	1 cup chicken with sauce + 1/2 cup cooked rice

This recipe is good for 4 servings.

You will need:

- 1 pound boneless chicken breast, skin removed and cut into 2-inch strips
- 2 tsp peanut oil
- 1 1/2 tbsps. cornstarch
- 2 cloves garlic, minced
- 1/2 tsp red pepper flakes
- 2 medium scallions, chopped
- 1/2 tsp ginger powder
- 1 tbsp. white wine vinegar
- 2 cups white rice, cooked and kept warm
- 2 tbsps. sugar
- 2 tbsps. low sodium soy sauce
- 3/4 cup canned chicken broth

How to do it:

Combine broth, sugar, soy sauce, ginger, vinegar, and cornstarch in a bowl. Set aside.

Heat wok over medium heat and add some oil. Stir in scallions, garlic, and red pepper flakes. Cook for 2 minutes. Stir in the chicken strips and cook for 5 minutes.

Pour the broth mixture into the pan. Simmer until the sauce thickens.

Italian Pesto Chicken Burger

Prep Time	:	10 minutes
Cook Time	:	15 minutes
Smart Points per serving	:	7
1 Serving	:	1 sandwich

This recipe is good for 2 servings.

You will need:

- 2 tsp reduced-fat pesto sauce
- 2 tsp fat-free mayonnaise
- 2 pieces chicken burgers
- 2 pieces light hamburger buns, toasted
- 2 leaves of romaine lettuce
- 1/2 cup red peppers, roasted and chopped
- 1/3 cup part-skim mozzarella cheese, grated
- 1 pinch each of salt and ground black pepper
- Cooking spray

How to do it:

Mix pesto and mayonnaise in a lidded bowl. Cover and put in a refrigerator.

Combine the salt and pepper and rub all over the burger patties. Spray some oil on the grill and preheat it. Grill the chicken until all sides are cooked.

Put cheese on top of the burger patty. Put mayonnaise-pesto mixture on each bun, followed by the lettuce. Add the grilled burger patty and peppers on each bun. Serve.

Taco Stuffed Chicken

Prep Time	:	15 minutes
Cook Time	:	20 minutes
Smart Points per serving	:	5
1 Serving	:	1 chicken breast cutlet

This recipe is good for 4 servings.

You will need:

- 4 pieces 5oz-breast cutlet, boneless skinless
- 15 pieces baked tortilla chips, crushed
- 4 wedges light creamy Swiss cheese
- 1/4 cup taco sauce
- 3 tbsps. thick salsa
- Salt and pepper to taste

How to do it:

Preheat oven to 350°F.

Coat an 8-inch x 8-inch baking dish with nonstick spray.

Mix cheese wedges in a bowl until smooth. Stir in salsa until well blended.

Pound the chicken cutlets into 1/3 inch thickness and season the cutlets with pepper and salt. Distribute the cheese mixture evenly among the cutlets. Make sure to put it in the center of each cutlet.

Tightly roll each cutlet and be careful not to let the cheese mixture ooze out. Secure the cutlet with a toothpick.

Arrange the cutlets in the baking dish. Cover it with foil and bake for 20 minutes.

Take the cutlets out of the oven. Spread 1 tablespoon taco sauce on each cutlet, then top with crushed tortilla chips. Put the cutlets back in the oven and bake until the chicken is cooked through.

Spinach and Feta Stuffed Chicken

Prep Time	:	15 minutes
Cook Time	:	45 minutes
Smart Points per serving	:	4
1 Serving	:	1 stuffed chicken

This recipe is good for 2 servings.

You will need:

- 2 pieces 5oz-chicken breast cutlet, skin removed
- 1/4 cup reduced-fat feta cheese, crumbled
- 2 cups spinach leaves, coarsely chopped
- 1 tsp garlic, minced
- Salt and black pepper to taste

How to do it:

Preheat oven to 350ºF. Coat an 8-inch x 8-inch baking dish with nonstick spray.

Put the spinach in a microwave-safe bowl and set the microwave for 30 seconds. Use a paper towel to absorb the excess moisture from the spinach. Add garlic and feta. Mix well.

Pound the chicken cutlets into 1/4 inch thickness and season with pepper and salt. Divide the cheese mixture evenly among the cutlets. Stuff it in the center of each cutlet.

Roll each cutlet and be careful not to let the mixture ooze out. Secure the cutlet with a toothpick. Do the same to the rest of the cutlets.

Place the cutlets in the baking dish. Put a foil over it and bake for 20 minutes.

Remove the cover and put the cutlets back in the oven. Bake until chicken is cooked through.

Kickin' Chicken Pot Pie

Prep Time	:	5 minutes
Cook Time	:	60 minutes
Smart Points per serving	:	7
1 Serving	:	1 portion

This recipe is good for 8 servings.

You will need:

- 1 pound boneless and skinless chicken breast, cut into bite-size pieces
- 1 package refrigerated Pillsbury Crescent Recipe Creations Seamless Dough Sheet
- 2 cans of fat-free cream of celery condensed soup (one can is about 10.75oz)
- 6 cups frozen mixed vegetables, thawed

How to do it:

Preheat oven to 350°F. Prepare a baking dish and coat it with cooking spray.

Put a large skillet with nonstick spray coating over medium heat. Add the chicken and stir-fry for about 10 to 15 minutes.

Transfer the cooked chicken to a large bowl. Add the soup and thawed vegetables. Combine well. Pour the mixture into the baking dish and put in the oven. Bake the chicken until the top becomes bubbly.

Put the dough sheet over the baking dish and stretch to cover the cooked chicken in the dish. Put it back in the oven and bake until the dough turns golden brown.

Cut it into 8 equal portions and serve.

Fajita-Stuffed Chicken

Prep Time	:	15 minutes
Cook Time	:	45 minutes
Smart Points per serving	:	4
1 Serving	:	1 chicken cutlet fajita + 2 tbsps. salsa

This recipe is good for 2 servings.

You will need:

- 2 pieces 5oz-chicken breast cutlet (skinless), pounded to half inch thickness
- 1/4 cup reduced-fat Mexican-blend cheese, shredded
- 1/2 cup onion, sliced
- 1/4 cup salsa
- 1/2 cup green and red bell peppers, sliced
- 2 tsp fajita seasoning mix
- Salt and black pepper

How to do it:

Preheat oven to 350°F. Coat a baking pan with nonstick spray.

Coat a skillet with nonstick spray and put it over medium heat. Add bell peppers and onion in the skillet and sauté for about 6 minutes.

Transfer the cooked bell peppers and onion in a medium bowl. Add a teaspoon of fajita seasoning, and mix well.

Season the chicken cutlets with the remaining fajita seasoning, salt, and black pepper. Divide the cooked veggies into 2 equal portions. Spread one portion of the cooked veggies to the center of each cutlet.

Roll up each cutlet and secure it. Arrange the stuffed cutlets in the baking dish. Cover it with foil and bake for 20 minutes.

Remove the foil, and sprinkle cheese over the stuffed cutlets. Bake until chicken is thoroughly cooked. Serve each cutlet with salsa.

Tandoori Chicken with Chutney

Prep Time	:	20 minutes
Cook Time	:	20 minutes
Smart Points per serving	:	7
1 Serving	:	1

This recipe is good for 4 servings.

You will need:

- 450g skinless chicken breast, cubed
- 2 garlic cloves, crushed
- 1 onion, coarsely chopped
- 1/2 green chili, coarsely chopped
- 1 two-cm fresh ginger, sliced
- 2 tsp garam masala
- 1/2 teaspoon ground turmeric
- 400g can chopped tomatoes
- 3 tbsps. tomato purée
- 200g fat-free natural yogurt
- 200ml gluten free chicken stock
- 200g dried brown rice
- salt and freshly ground black pepper
- calorie controlled cooking spray

Ingredients you will need for the Green Chutney:

- 4 tbsps. chopped fresh coriander
- 2 tbsps. fresh mint, chopped
- Half green chili
- 1/2 lime, get the juice
- 2 tbsps. fat-free natural Yogurt

How to do it:

Put the ginger, garlic, onion, chili, and spices in a blender to make a paste. Add 4 tablespoons of water and seasoning. Transfer to a bowl and set aside.

Prepare the brown rice and cook according to the direction in the package.

Get a non-stick frying pan and coat with cooking spray. Pour in the paste mixture and cook for 4 to 5 minutes. Stir the mixture constantly until the paste becomes a bit dry and fragrant. Stir in the tomato puree and cook for 1 minute. Transfer to a plate to cool.

Get a non-reactive container and combine half of the paste and yogurt. Add the chicken. Cover the container and marinate for 2 hours or overnight in the refrigerator. Chill the rest of the paste.

When everything is ready, preheat the grill. Pour the chilled curry paste into a saucepan. Add the chopped tomatoes and chicken stock. Cover the pan and simmer for 15 minutes.

Arrange the marinated chicken on a foil-lined tray, and grill for about 10 minutes or until the chicken is cooked through. Drop the Tandoori chicken into the curry sauce and cook for 3 to 4 minutes.

Combine all the ingredients for the chutney in a blender. Scoop some rice on the plate with chicken in curry sauce. Pour some chutney on the chicken.

Serve and enjoy.

Chinese Chicken Salad

Prep Time	:	10 minutes
Cook Time	:	n/a
Smart Points per serving	:	5
1 Serving	:	1/4 of the recipe

This recipe is good for 4 servings.

You will need:

- 12oz skinless lean chicken breast, pre-cooked and chopped
- 1 cup scallions, chopped
- 3/4 cup sesame ginger dressing (choose low-fat)
- 1 cup water chestnuts, sliced and drained
- 1 cup mandarin orange segments in can, chopped
- 5 1/2 cups broccoli, dry slaw

How to do it:

Get a casserole and combine chicken, slaw, orange, water chestnuts, and scallions. Mix well. Add the dressing and mix everything to coat well.

BBQ Chicken Quesadilla

Prep Time	:	10 minutes
Cook Time	:	5 minutes
Smart Points per serving	:	8
1 Serving	:	1 quesadilla

This recipe is good for 4 servings.

You will need:

- 2oz skinless chicken breast, pre-cooked and shredded
- 1 tbsp. scallions, chopped
- 1 wedge light creamy Swiss cheese
- 2 tbsps. reduced-fat Mexican-blend cheese, shredded
- 1 medium to large high-fiber flour tortilla
- 1 tbsp. frozen sweet corn kernels, thawed
- 1 tbsp. canned black beans, rinsed and drained
- 1 tbsp. low calorie BBQ sauce

How to do it:

Combine cheese wedge and BBQ sauce in a bowl. Mix thoroughly until smooth. Spread the tortilla on a flat surface. Spread the cheese mixture on half of the tortilla. Add the remaining ingredients on top of the mixture.

Coat the grill pan with nonstick spray and put it over medium heat. Put the tortilla with the mixture in the grill pan and cook for 2 minutes.

Gently fold the other half of the tortilla over the side with filling. Press lightly to seal. Flip the quesadilla and cook for 3 minutes more. Slice into wedges and enjoy.

Fish Recipes

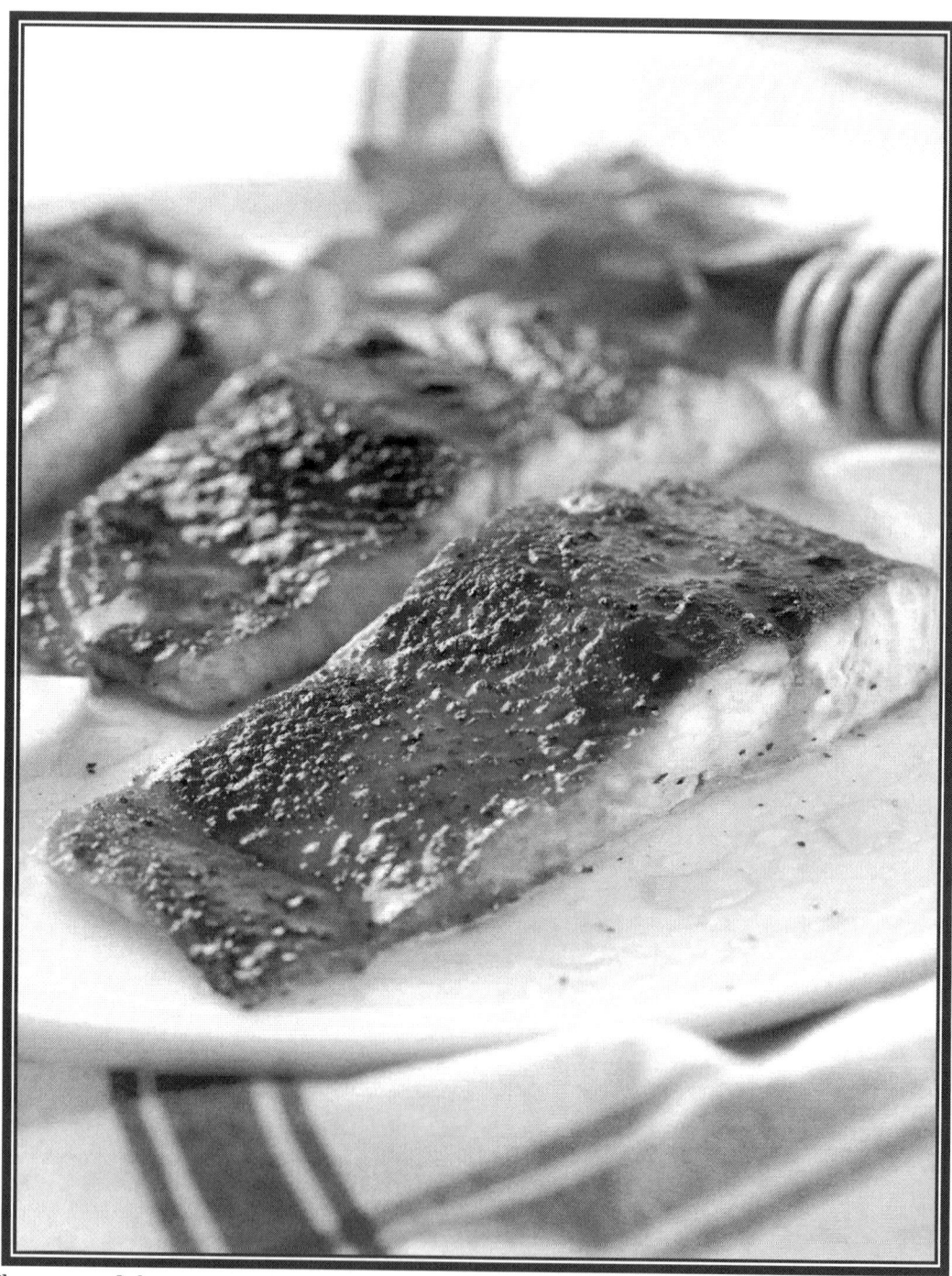

These tasty fish recipes will make you come back for more.

Roasted Salmon in Honey-Mustard

Prep Time	:	12 minutes
Cook Time	:	18 minutes
Smart Points per serving	:	6
1 Serving	:	1 6oz-fillet + mustard sauce

This recipe is good for 4 servings.

You will need:

- 4 pieces of 6oz-fillet pink salmon
- 1/4 tsp garlic powder
- 1 tbsp. vinegar (from white wine)
- 1/4 tsp dry mustard
- 1/4 cup mustard (Dijon)
- 2 tsp fresh dill, chopped
- 1 tbsp. water
- 2 tbsps. honey
- 1/8 tsp each of salt and black pepper
- Cooking spray

How to do it:

Prepare a baking pan and smear it with oil spray.

Rub pepper and salt to the fish fillets and arrange them in the baking dish.

Whisk the dry mustard, honey, vinegar, garlic powder, Dijon mustard, and water in a bowl. Set aside some mustard sauce (about 2 tablespoons), and use it to rub all over the salmon fillets. Add the dill into the rest of the mustard sauce.

Roast the salmon in the oven at 400 ºF until cooked. Put some mustard sauce on top and serve.

Spicy BBQ Salmon and Veggies

Prep Time	:	10 minutes
Cook Time	:	20 minutes
Smart Points per serving	:	9
1 Serving	:	1 salmon fillet

This recipe is good for 1 serving.

You will need:

- 4oz salmon fillet, skin removed
- 1 cup broccoli, cut into florets
- Half cup yellow squash, chopped
- 2 tbsps. low-calorie BBQ sauce
- 1/2 cup zucchini, chopped
- 1 tsp Sriracha

How to do it:

Get a baking sheet and line it with foil. Coat the foil with cooking spray.

Mix Sriracha and BBQ sauce in a bowl until well blended.

Put the vegetables in the middle of the foil. Place the salmon on top and smear with the prepared mixture. Cut another foil to cover the top.

Crimp the edges of the foil to seal the salmon. Put it in a 375°F oven and bake for 20 minutes.

Let it cool for a bit. Open and serve.

Grilled Salmon with Mustard

Prep Time	:	8 minutes
Cook Time	:	12 minutes
Smart Points per serving	:	7
1 Serving	:	5 ounces salmon + 1 1/2 tbsps. sauce

This recipe is good for 4 servings.

You will need:

- 20oz fresh salmon fillets, skin removed and cut equally into 4
- 3 tbsps. fresh thyme, chopped
- 3 tbsps. rosemary, chopped
- 1 tsp black pepper, freshly ground
- 4 tbsps. Dijon Mustard
- Cooking spray

How to do it:

Combine pepper, thyme, and rosemary in a bowl.

Coat the peeled off part of the fish with cooking spray.

Get a tablespoon of mustard and spread it on top of each fillet. Get 1 1/2 tablespoons herb mixture and sprinkle it next.

Arrange the fish on the grill. Make sure to place the part with oil on the grill. Cover the grill and cook for about 12 minutes.

Transfer the cooked fish to a serving platter.

Grilled Yellowfin Tuna with Teriyaki Sauce

Prep Time	:	8 minutes
Cook Time	:	9 minutes
Smart Points per serving	:	6
1 Serving	:	3 ounces tuna

This recipe is good for 4 servings.

You will need:

- 16oz yellowfin tuna, sliced to 1-inch thickness
- 1 tbsp. cornstarch
- 1 tbsp. sherry cooking wine
- 3 cloves garlic, minced
- 3 tbsps. packed brown sugar
- 2 tbsps. ginger, finely chopped
- 1/2 cup low sodium soy sauce
- 1/2 cup unsweetened orange juice
- 1/4 cup water
- Cooking spray

How to do it:

Spray some oil on the grill and preheat it.

To make a teriyaki sauce, mix soy sauce, sherry, ginger, garlic, water, orange juice, cornstarch, and sugar in a saucepan. Stir constantly and bring to a boil.

Once the sauce becomes thick, you can turn off the stove. Spread the teriyaki sauce all over the fish. Grill the fish until all sides are cooked.

Grilled Fish with Tartar Sauce

Prep Time	:	20 minutes
Cook Time	:	8 minutes
Smart Points per serving	:	4
1 Serving	:	1 piece of halibut + tartar sauce

This recipe is good for 6 servings.

You will need:

- 2 pounds halibut fillets, cut into 6 equal pieces
- 1/4 cup onion, finely chopped
- 1 tbsp. fresh parsley, finely chopped
- 2 tbsps. fresh dill, finely chopped
- 2 tbsps. fresh lemon juice
- 1/4 cup unsweetened dill pickles, finely chopped
- 1 tbsp. olive oil
- 1/4 cup light mayonnaise
- 2 tbsps. capers, finely chopped
- 1/2 tsp sugar
- Salt and pepper to taste
- Cooking spray

How to do it:

Combine a tablespoon of lemon juice and oil in a cup. Rub each fillet with the mixture and arrange them in a glass dish. Refrigerate the covered dish.

To make a tartar sauce, you need to combine pickles, dill, onion, capers, parsley, lemon juice, pepper, sugar, and salt in a bowl. Stir in the mayonnaise. Set aside.

Cover the grill with cooking spray and preheat it. Grill each side of the fish for 4 minutes. Serve with tartar sauce.

Grilled Trout with Stuffed Oregano and Lemon

Prep Time	:	10 minutes
Cook Time	:	14 minutes
Smart Points per serving	:	3
1 Serving	:	3 ounces of trout

This recipe is good for 4 servings.

You will need:

- 2 pieces 8oz-trout, boneless
- 1/2 lemon, sliced into thin half-moons
- 8 sprigs fresh oregano
- 1/2 lemon, squeeze the juice
- Salt and pepper to taste
- Cooking spray

How to do it:

Cover the grill with cooking spray and preheat it.

Rub salt and pepper all over the trout. Put 4 sprigs of oregano and half the lemon slices inside each trout.

Grill the trout until cooked. Splash some lemon juice on the trout while grilling. Make sure to cook each side evenly.

Vegetable Recipes

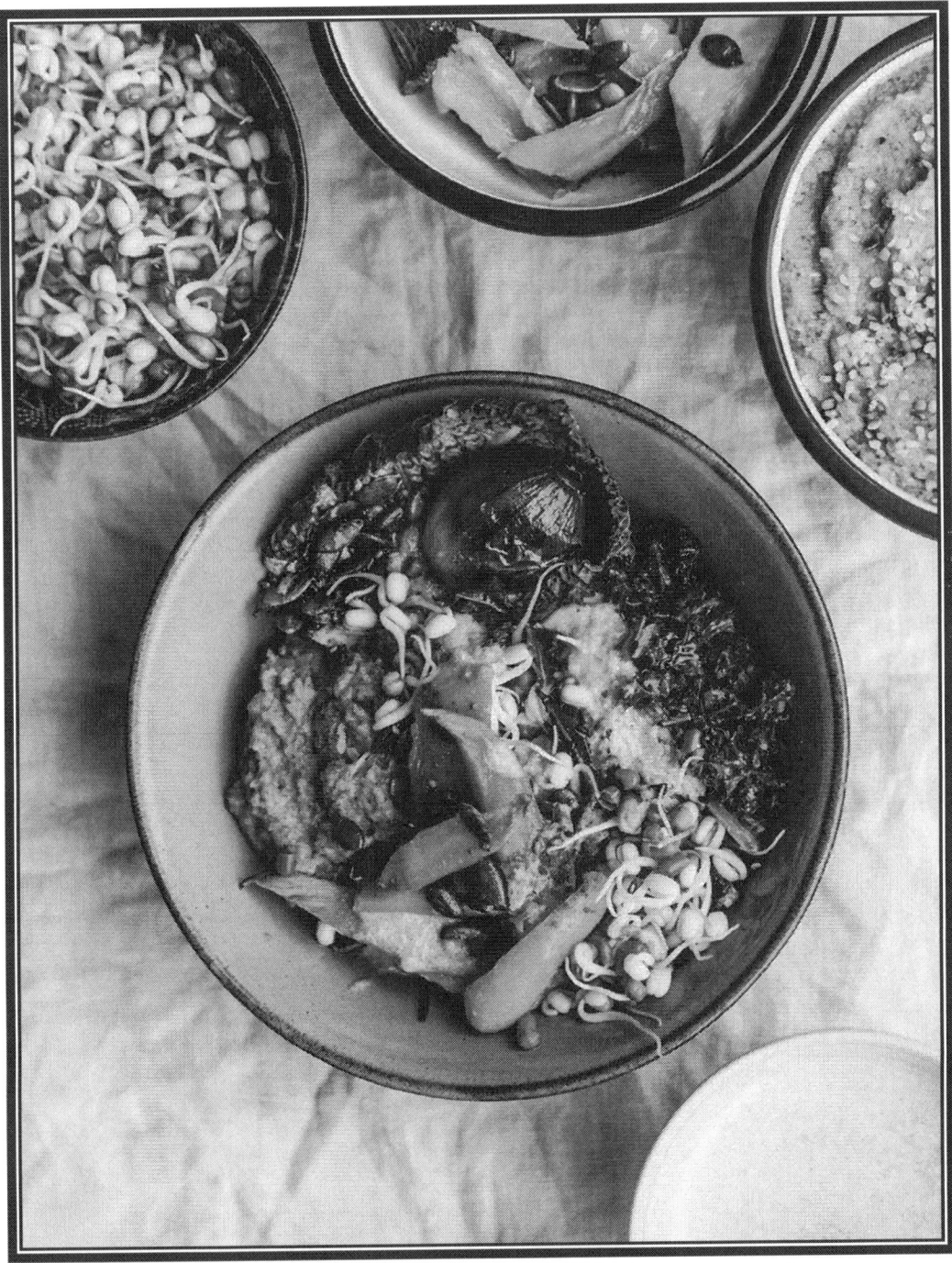

These vegetable recipes are packed with flavor and all the important nutrients.

Barley-Asparagus Risotto with Balsamic Vinegar

Prep Time	:	15 minutes
Cook Time	:	20 minutes
Smart Points per serving	:	5
1 Serving	:	About 1 cup

This recipe is good for 6 servings.

You will need:

- 1/2 pound asparagus, trimmed and cut into 2-inch pieces
- 1 medium onion, chopped
- 1/4 cup chives, sliced
- 1 cup pearl barley, choose the quick-cooking variety
- 2 tsp olive oil
- 3 cups fat-free chicken or vegetable broth
- 2 tbsps. grated Parmesan cheese
- 1 1/2 tbsps. balsamic vinegar
- 1/8 tsp salt
- 1/8 tsp black pepper, freshly ground

How to do it:

Put a large saucepan over medium heat. Add some oil when the saucepan is hot. Add in onion. Stir until the onion becomes tender. Add barley. Continue stirring and cook for another minute.

Pour in the broth, cover, and let it simmer for 8 minutes over low heat. Add the asparagus and simmer for 2 minutes.

Remove from heat, add the chives and vinegar. Season with salt and pepper. Sprinkle some cheese and serve.

Baked Vegetable Tart

Prep Time	:	35 minutes
Cook Time	:	105 minutes
Smart Points per serving	:	9
1 Serving	:	1/6 of Vegetable Tart

This recipe is good for 6 servings.

You will need:

- 600g orange sweet potato
- 1 large fresh eggplant
- 1 medium red onion
- 2 medium zucchinis
- 1 tbsp. olive oil
- 2 medium red capsicums
- 1/4 cup fresh basil, slightly crushed
- 8 medium eggs, lightly beaten
- 8 sheets filo pastry
- 1 tbsp. pine nuts, toasted
- 2 tbsps. parmesan cheese, grated
- Cooking spray

How to do it:

Preheat oven to 350°F.

Slice the red onion, capsicum, eggplant, sweet potato, and zucchini into 3cm pieces.

Prepare 2 baking trays. Line each tray with baking paper. Put the eggplant, onion, capsicum, and sweet potato in the trays. Spray some oil, toss, and season with salt and pepper. Bake for 1 hour.

Prepare a 22cm pie dish with a removable base and spray it with oil. Place 1 sheet of pastry on a flat surface and spray some oil. Place another sheet on the first sheet on a 45-degree angle, and spray some oil. Repeat the procedure until you have no more filo left. Arrange the piled pastry in the pie dish. Fold the overhanging filo in the dish.

Arrange the vegetables in the dish and sprinkle some parmesan. Add the eggs. Put the pie dish on a baking sheet. Bake for 45 to 50 minutes. Add pine nuts and basil on top. Slice into 6 equal parts.

Cellophane Noodles with Garlic, Cilantro, and Cucumbers

Prep Time	:	30 minutes
Cook Time	:	7 minutes
Smart Points per serving	:	5
1 Serving	:	1 1/2 cups

This recipe is good for 4 servings.

You will need:

- 3 3/4oz cellophane noodles
- 1 1/2 tbsps. fish sauce
- 1 cup snow peas, julienne cut
- 1/2 cup fresh cilantro, coarsely chopped
- 3 cloves garlic, minced
- 2 medium carrots, julienne cut
- 1 tbsp. vegetable oil
- 1 medium cucumber, julienne cut
- 1/4 cup rice wine vinegar
- 1 tbsp. sugar

How to do it:

Pour water in a large pot and bring it to a boil. Drop the noodles and simmer for 3 minutes. Drain and set aside.

Mix garlic, cilantro, sugar, vinegar, oil, and fish sauce in a casserole. Add noodles, cucumber, snow peas, and carrots. Toss well.

Grilled BBQ Tempeh

Prep Time	:	10 minutes
Cook Time	:	30 minutes
Smart Points per serving	:	10
1 Serving	:	4 slices tempeh + 1/4 cup onions

This recipe is good for 4 servings.

You will need:

- 10oz tempeh, cut into 16 pieces
- 1 medium onion, sliced
- 1 cup barbecue sauce
- 1 tsp sesame oil

How to do it:

Arrange the tempeh slices in a steamer and put it over medium heat. Steam the tempeh for about 20 minutes. Set aside

Get a pan and put it over medium heat. Add sesame oil and sauté the onion.

Preheat the grill. Brush the barbecue sauce on tempeh slices and grill each side for 5 minutes. Don't forget to brush the tempeh with the sauce as you grill.

Bok Choy and Tofu Stir-Fry

Prep Time	:	20 minutes
Cook Time	:	5 minutes
Smart Points per serving	:	5
1 Serving	:	1 cup tofu mixture + 1/2 cup rice

This recipe is good for 4 servings.

You will need:

- 4 cups bok choy, coarsely chopped
- 1 cup dried shiitake mushroom caps, sliced
- 1 small piece ginger root, grated
- 2 tbsps. hoisin sauce
- 12oz tofu, cut into half-inch cubes
- 1 clove garlic, minced
- 2 tbsps. low sodium soy sauce
- 1/4 cup scallion, chopped
- 1/4 tsp black pepper
- 2 cups brown rice, cooked
- Cooking spray

How to do it:

Cover the wok or skillet with cooking spray. Put it over medium heat. Stir-fry mushrooms, ginger, garlic, and bok choy for about 3 minutes. Add tofu cubes and fry each side until it turns golden brown.

Stir in hoisin sauce, scallions, pepper, and soy sauce. Cook for 1 minute. Serve.

California Club Wrap

Prep Time	:	8 minutes
Cook Time	:	0 minutes
Smart Points per serving	:	4
1 Serving	:	1 California club wrap

This recipe is good for 1 serving.

You will need:

- 1 medium fat-free flour tortilla
- 1/4 small cucumber, thinly sliced
- 2 tbsps. store-bought hummus
- 1 small fresh tomato, thinly sliced
- 1/2 cup fresh watercress, cut off the thick stems
- Salt and black pepper to taste

Procedure:

Spread the tortilla on a flat surface. Smear some hummus on the tortilla. Spread the tomatoes, cucumber, and watercress. Sprinkle some salt and pepper to taste. Roll the tortilla and enjoy.

Greek-Style Spaghetti Squash

Prep Time		:	20 minutes
Cook Time		:	25 minutes
Smart Points per serving		:	2
1 Serving		:	1 cup squash mixture + 1 tbsp. cheese

This recipe is good for 4 servings.

You will need:

- 2 pounds spaghetti squash
- 1/2 cup scallions, sliced
- 1/4 cup pot cheese or fat-free crumbled feta
- 2 tsp olive oil
- 1 cup chickpeas, drained and rinsed
- 2 tsp garlic, minced
- 14 1/2oz can diced tomatoes, do not drain
- 1 tsp dried oregano
- 1 tsp lemon zest, grated
- 1/4 cup dill, chopped
- 1/4 tsp table salt
- 1/4 tsp black pepper

How to do the squash spaghetti strands:

Preheat oven to 350ºF.

Wash the squash and cut it in half, lengthwise. Scoop out the seeds. Prepare a baking dish and coat it with nonstick spray. Put the squash in the baking dish, cut side down.

Prick the squash all over using a fork. Put in the oven and bake for about 30 to 40 minutes or until tender.

Use a fork to scrape the squash and produce the spaghetti strands. Set aside.

How to do the recipe:

Get a large nonstick skillet and put it over medium heat. Add some oil and sauté garlic and scallions for about a minute. Add lemon zest, chickpeas, tomatoes, pepper, oregano, and salt. Turn the heat to high and bring to a boil.

Add the squash spaghetti strands in the skillet. Stir well until the squash strands are thoroughly coated with the mixture. Turn off the stove and add the dill into the spaghetti. Top it with cheese when served.

Tomato-Basil Sauce Eggplant Involtini

Prep Time	:	28 minutes
Cook Time	:	42 minutes
Smart Points per serving	:	3
1 Serving	:	2 pieces of involtini

This recipe is good for 4 servings.

You will need:

- 2 medium eggplants
- 1 tsp olive oil
- 4 cloves of large garlic, minced
- 1 medium onion, finely chopped
- 2 tbsps. fresh basil, torn
- 2 tbsps. fresh basil, chopped
- 2 cups canned tomatoes, crushed
- 1 large egg
- 1/2 cup part-skim ricotta cheese
- 1 small zucchini, diced
- 1/2 cup fresh parsley, chopped
- 3 tbsps. Parmesan cheese, grated
- 1/4 tsp table salt
- 1/4 tsp black pepper, ground
- Cooking spray

How to do it:

Preheat oven to 450ºF. Spray some oil on a baking sheet.

Remove the top and bottom of each eggplant. Slice the eggplants lengthwise into 4 equal parts.

Arrange the eggplant slices on the baking sheet. Make sure that no eggplant slice overlaps with another. Lightly coat the eggplant slices with cooking spray. Bake the eggplant for 10 minutes, flip them once and continue baking for another 10 minutes. Remove from the oven and set aside.

To make the sauce, put a saucepan over medium heat. Add oil. Stir in half of the minced garlic and sauté for 1 to 2 minutes. Stir in the crushed tomatoes and torn basil to combine. Reduce heat and simmer for 10 minutes. Turn off the stove, cover the pan, and set aside.

To make the filling, spray some oil on a large nonstick skillet. Put it over medium heat. Add the onion and zucchini and sauté for about 5 minutes. Add the remaining garlic and cook for another minute. Transfer it to a bowl. Get another bowl and combine the chopped basil, ricotta, 2 tablespoons parmesan, and parsley. Add the onion mixture and blend well. Stir in egg, pepper, and salt.

To make the involtini, preheat oven to 400ºF. Prepare an 8-inch x 8-inch baking dish. Put 3 tablespoons of sauce in the dish and swirl to cover the entire bottom. Get a clean cutting board and place a slice of eggplant on top.

Get 3 tablespoons of sauce and spread at the bottom of a baking pan, coat well. On a clean surface, place 1 slice of eggplant. Spread 2 tablespoons of filling at the tapered end of the eggplant slice. Roll it up and secure it with a toothpick if needed. Do the same with the rest of the eggplant slices. Arrange the involtinis in the baking dish. Smear the remaining sauce and parmesan cheese over them. Bake for about 10 to 15 minutes.

Grilled Vegetables and Haloumi

Prep Time	:	10 minutes
Cook Time	:	5 minutes
Smart Points per serving	:	7
1 Serving	:	1 slice bread + 1/4 of vegetables + 1/2 tsp pesto + 30g haloumi

This recipe is good for 4 servings.

You will need:

- 4 pieces of rye bread (around 40g per piece), toasted
- 120g halloumi cheese, cut into 1cm-thick strips
- 1 tbsp. pesto sauce
- 4 whole fresh mushrooms, trimmed
- 2 bunches of fresh asparagus, trimmed and halved
- 250g fresh cherry tomato
- Cooking spray

How to do it:

Preheat grill over medium fire. Coat the asparagus, tomatoes, halloumi, and mushrooms with cooking spray. Grill for about 3 or 4 minutes. Make sure that each side of halloumi turns golden brown.

Serve halloumi with toasted bread, pesto, and grilled vegetables.

Artichoke and Red Pepper Frittata

Prep Time	:	20 minutes
Cook Time	:	16 minutes
Smart Points per serving	:	5
1 Serving	:	1 slice

This recipe is good for 4 servings.

You will need:

- 6oz-can artichoke hearts (in water), coarsely chopped
- 1 cup red peppers, roasted and coarsely chopped
- 1/2 cup hard or semi-soft cheese, shredded
- 1 medium onion, chopped
- 1 medium potato, boiled and thickly sliced
- 1/2 tsp dried oregano
- 6 large egg whites
- 2 large whole eggs
- 1/2 tsp red pepper flakes, crushed
- 1/2 tsp salt
- 1/2 tsp black pepper
- Cooking spray

How to do it:

Cover a 10-inch nonstick skillet with oil and put it over medium heat.

Add the onion, peppers, artichokes, and potatoes in the skillet and sauté for 2 minutes.

Get a bowl and beat the egg whites and whole eggs. Add salt, red pepper flakes, oregano, and pepper. Pour the egg mixture over the vegetable mixture. Cook everything for 5 minutes. You need to lift the egg mixture to allow the raw eggs to run to the bottom of the skillet.

Sprinkle some cheese and place the skillet in a broiler. It is ready when the cheese has melted. Cut into 4 equal portions and serve.

Eggplant Parmigiana

Prep Time	:	15 minutes
Cook Time	:	35 minutes
Smart Points per serving	:	3
1 Serving	:	1/4 of Eggplant Parmigiana or 1 portion

This recipe is good for 4 servings.

You will need:

- 1 medium eggplant
- 1/4 tsp garlic powder
- 1/3 cup seasoned bread crumbs, Italian-style
- 1 tbsp. Parmesan cheese, grated
- 1/2 cup part-skim mozzarella cheese, shredded
- 1 tsp Italian seasoning
- 2 egg whites, lightly beaten
- 1 1/2 cups tomato sauce
- Cooking spray

How to do it:

Preheat oven to 350°F.

Prepare a 9 x 13-inch baking dish and coat it with cooking spray.

Combine the garlic powder, bread crumbs, Italian seasoning, and Parmesan cheese in a bowl. Peel off the eggplant skin and trim off its ends. Slice the eggplant into 1/2-inch thickness.

Dip the eggplant slices in the egg whites and then the breadcrumb mixture. Place the eggplant slices on a nonstick baking sheet. Bake for about 20 to 25 minutes, flip them once.

Arrange a layer of eggplant slices at the bottom of the baking dish. Add 1/3 each of tomato sauce and mozzarella cheese. Repeat the same procedure with 2 more layers, don't alter the order. Bake until the sauce becomes bubbly. Slice into 4 equal portions and serve.

Caramelized Onion and Mushroom Lasagna

Prep Time	:	28 minutes
Cook Time	:	65 minutes
Smart Points per serving	:	9
1 Serving	:	1 slice

This recipe is good for 8 servings.

You will need:

- 3/4 pound lasagna noodles, cook according to package direction
- 6 medium Portobello mushrooms
- 1/2 pound cremini mushrooms
- 3 cloves garlic, minced
- 2 large onions, peeled and thickly sliced
- 1 tbsp. olive oil
- 2 tbsps. olive oil
- 1/2 tsp nutmeg, freshly grated
- 1 tbsp. fresh rosemary, chopped
- 1/2 cup water
- 1/4 cup diet cola
- 3 tbsps. all-purpose flour
- 1 tbsp. salted butter
- 1/4 cup Parmesan cheese, grated
- 3 cups fat-free skim milk
- 1/2 tsp table salt
- Cooking spray

How to do it:

Remove the stems from the mushrooms and cut the caps into 1/4 inch-thick slices. Set aside.

Put a large nonstick skillet over medium heat. Add oil and onions. Let the onions caramelize for 3 minutes before stirring it occasionally for the next 7 minutes. Stir in rosemary and let it released its flavor before pouring in water. Cook for about 2 to 3 minutes to reduce the water. Add soda and cook until onions are soft with a nice touch of brown. Transfer to a large bowl and set aside.

Spray some oil on the same skillet and put over medium heat. Add mushrooms and cook for about 2 to 3 minutes, don't stir. Season with salt and stir the mushrooms occasionally for about 3 to 4 minutes. Add the cooked mushrooms to the bowl of onions.

Preheat oven to 350ºF.

To make the sauce: put the same skillet over medium heat. Add remaining oil and melt butter. Stir in flour and mix until combined. Pour in milk, a little at a time, while stirring constantly to avoid the formation of lumps. Bring to a boil. Add in garlic and continue to cook while stirring for about 3 to 4 minutes. Add 2 tablespoons of cheese and nutmeg. Continue to stir until well blended. Set aside.

To assemble: prepare a 9-inch x 11-inch baking dish and coat the bottom with 1/3 cup sauce. Add 3 lasagna noodles to cover the sauce. Spread 1/3 cup of sauce and 1 1/2 cups of the onion-mushroom mixture over the lasagna noodles. Add another 1/4 cup sauce. Cover the sauce with 3 lasagna noodles. Repeat the same process, ending it with 1/4 cup sauce. For the finishing touch, sprinkle the remaining cheese on top.

Put it in the oven and bake for 20 minutes. Turn the oven temperature to broil and cook until the lasagna top becomes crispy. Take it out of the oven and let it cool for a bit before slicing it into eight equal slices.

Baked Pasta with Butternut Squash

Prep Time	:	25 minutes
Cook Time	:	60 minutes
Smart Points per serving	:	6
1 Serving	:	1 cup

This recipe is good for 8 servings.

You will need:

- 20oz butternut squash, peeled and cubed
- 1 tbsp. fresh thyme, chopped
- 2 tsp garlic, minced
- 1/4 tbsp. walnuts, toasted and chopped
- 12 oz. whole wheat penne pasta
- 1 1/4 cups fat-free skim milk
- 1/3 cup Parmesan cheese, grated
- 2 tbsps. white all-purpose flour
- 1/2 cup part-skim ricotta cheese
- 1/2 tsp salt
- 1/4 tsp black pepper, ground
- Cooking spray

How to do it:

Preheat oven to 375ºF. Spray some oil on a baking sheet and place the squash. Put the baking sheet with squash in the oven and roast for about 20 to 30 minutes. Transfer the roasted squash to a large bowl and mash.

Prepare to cook the pasta according to package directions. Drain the pasta and put it back in the pot.

Get a medium saucepan and combine flour, milk, garlic, pepper, and salt. Bring to a boil while whisking frequently. Bring the heat to low and let it simmer while stirring for about 2 minutes.

Remove the flour mixture from heat. Set aside a half teaspoon of thyme for later and add the mashed squash and the rest of thyme into the flour mixture. Pour the sauce over the pasta. Toss to coat well.

Prepare a 3-quart baking dish and coat it with cooking spray. Transfer the pasta mixture into the baking dish. Scatter the ricotta on top and sprinkle with walnuts and parmesan. Bake for about 15 to 20 minutes. Remove from oven and sprinkle the half teaspoon of thyme on top.

Chickpea and Brown Rice Veggie Burgers with Tomato Salad

Prep Time	:	25 minutes
Cook Time	:	16 minutes
Smart Points per serving	:	4
1 Serving	:	1 burger + 1/4 cup salad

This recipe is good for 4 servings.

You will need:

- 1/2 cup brown rice, cooked
- 1 cup chickpeas, drained and rinsed
- 3 tbsps. shredded carrots
- 3 tbsps. scallions, finely chopped
- 2 tbsps. dried plain breadcrumbs
- 2 tbsps. fresh parsley, chopped
- 1 tsp lemon zest
- 1 tbsp. fresh cilantro, chopped
- 1 tsp coriander, ground
- 1/2 tsp salt
- 1/4 tsp black pepper, ground

Things you will need for the salad:

- 2 tbsps. red onion, thinly sliced
- 1 small cucumber, diced
- 2 tbsps. fresh parsley, chopped
- 3 tbsps. fresh lemon juice
- 1/4 cup sweet red peppers, diced
- 1 large egg white
- 1/4 cup cherry tomatoes, quartered
- 1 tbsp. extra-virgin olive oil
- 1/4 tsp salt
- 1/4 tsp black pepper, ground

How to do it:

Drop the chickpeas in a food processor and pulse using 10-second intervals. Aim for a coarse texture. Add in rice and pulse for another 10 seconds to combine.

Transfer the chickpea-rice mixture into a large bowl. Add lemon zest, carrots, parsley, cilantro, bread crumbs, coriander, scallion, salt, and pepper. Mix well to combine. Fold in egg white and mix gently to combine. Refrigerate the mixture for 10 minutes or overnight.

Get a medium bowl and combine all the ingredients for the salad. Set aside.

Spray some oil on the grill pan and preheat it over medium-high heat.

Divide the chickpea-rice mixture into 4 equal portions. Turn each portion into a patty. Coat the top part of each burger with cooking spray.

Grill one side of the burgers for about 6 to 8 minutes. Flip each burger and cook the other side for 6 to 8 minutes. Serve burgers with salad.

Soup Recipes

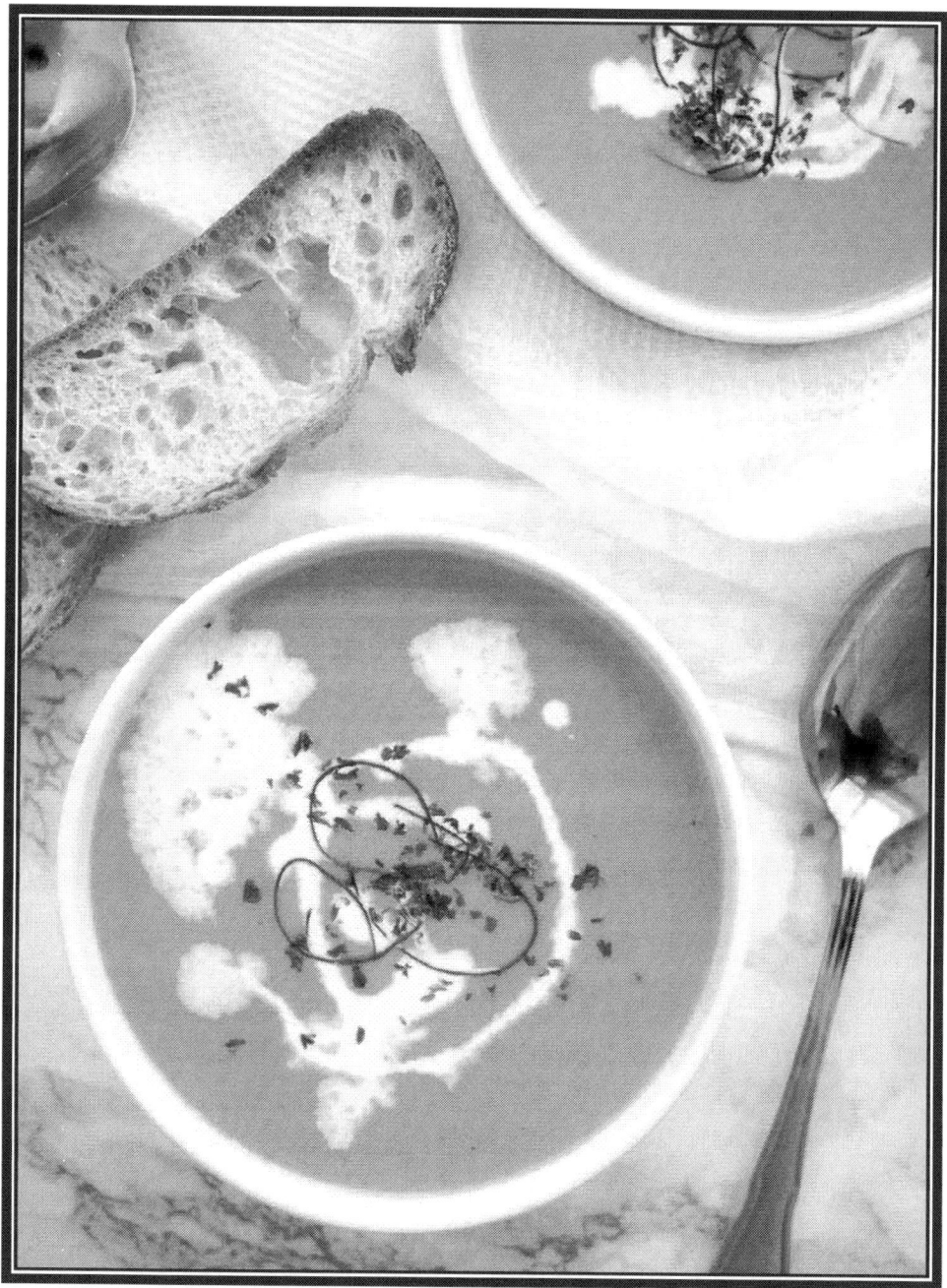

You will surely appreciate the different soup recipes in this chapter.

Zero Hero Soup

Prep Time	:	15 minutes
Cook Time	:	35 minutes
Smart Points per serving	:	0
1 Serving	:	1/6 of the soup

This recipe is good for 6 servings.

You will need:

- 1 large onion, chopped
- 1 tbsp. fresh parsley, chopped
- 2 large carrots, cubed
- 1 large zucchini, cubed
- 2 ribs of celery, sliced thinly
- 1 tsp dried mixed herbs
- 1 turnip, cubed
- 1.5 liters water
- 1 leek, sliced
- 2 vegetable stock cubes
- Salt and freshly ground black pepper

How to do it:

Pour water in a large saucepan and put it over high heat. Drop the crumbled stock cubes and bring to a boil. Stir it occasionally.

Add leek, onion, celery, zucchini, carrots, turnip. Stir in parsley and dried herbs. Let it boil for a while before reducing the heat. Simmer for 20 to 25 minutes and season with salt and pepper.

Cream of Broccoli Soup

Prep Time	:	14 minutes
Cook Time	:	20 minutes
Smart Points per serving	:	2
1 Serving	:	1 3/4 cups

This recipe is good for 4 servings.

You will need:

- 2 pounds broccoli, cut into florets
- 4 cups fat-free chicken or vegetable broth
- 1 medium onion, chopped
- 1 clove garlic, minced
- 1/4 cup water
- 1/2 tsp hot pepper sauce
- 1 cup evaporated milk
- Salt and pepper to taste

How to do it:

Boil the water with onion and garlic in a large soup pot. Bring down the heat and simmer for about 10 minutes. Stir in broccoli and broth to the pot and bring to a boil.

Bring down the heat and let it simmer for 8 minutes in the uncovered pot. Remove the soup from heat.

Prepare your blender. Pour the soup into the blender and puree until smooth. You may need to do it in batches. Transfer the pureed soup in a pot and stir in evaporated milk and hot pepper sauce, and season with salt and pepper.

Italian-Inspired Vegetable Soup

Prep Time	:	30 minutes
Cook Time	:	20 minutes
Smart Points per serving	:	0
1 Serving	:	1 cup

This recipe is good for 12 servings.

You will need:

- 2 small zucchinis, cubed
- 6 cups reduced sodium vegetable broth
- 28oz can tomatoes, fire-roasted and diced
- 1 tsp fresh oregano, finely chopped
- 2 cups fresh spinach baby leaves
- 2 cloves garlic, minced
- 1 medium fennel bulb, thinly sliced
- 1 cup onion, chopped
- 1/4 cup fresh basil leaves, torn
- 2 cups escarole, chopped
- 1/4 cup fresh parsley, chopped
- 2 tsp fresh thyme, finely chopped
- 1/4 tsp crushed red pepper flakes
- 1 medium sweet red pepper, chopped
- 3/4 tsp salt
- 1/4 tsp black pepper

How to do it:

Put all the ingredients in a large pot, except basil and parsley. Cover the pot, put it over high heat, and bring to a boil.

Reduce to low heat and simmer for 10 minutes.

Uncover the pot and stir in parsley and basil.

Super Easy Chicken Noodle Soup

Prep Time	:	12 minutes
Cook Time	:	20 minutes
Smart Points per serving	:	3
1 Serving	:	1 1/2 cups

This recipe is good for 8 servings.

You will need:

- 6oz skinless and boneless chicken breasts, cooked and coarsely chopped
- 1 large onion, finely chopped
- 15oz tomatoes, diced
- 10oz frozen mixed vegetables
- 2 tsp salted butter
- 4oz pasta, choose the small ones
- 64oz reduced-sodium chicken broth
- 2 tsp fresh lemon juice
- 1 tbsp. Parmesan cheese, grated
- 1 1/2 tsp salt
- 1/4 tsp black pepper

How to do it:

Prepare a large stockpot and put it over medium-low heat. Melt the butter in the pot. Stir in onion and sauté. Add 1/2 teaspoon salt and continue to stir.

Add the broth in the pot and bring to a boil. Drop the pasta, frozen vegetables, and tomatoes. Simmer until pasta becomes tender.

Add the chicken, cheese, salt, lemon juice, and pepper. Cook for a minute more and serve.

Veggie Soup

Prep Time	:	15 minutes
Cook Time	:	20 minutes
Smart Points per serving	:	0
1 Serving	:	1 cup

This recipe is good for 6 servings.

You will need:

- 1 medium red capsicum
- 2 pieces medium carrot
- 2 pieces medium zucchini
- 2 cloves fresh garlic, minced
- 4 cups chicken stock
- 1 medium onion, coarsely chopped
- 2 ribs of celery, trimmed and sliced
- 800g tomatoes in can, diced
- 1/3 cup fresh parsley
- 1/2 cup fresh basil

How to do it:

Cut the carrots, capsicums, and zucchinis into 1 cm slices.

Drop all the ingredients, except basil and parsley, into a large pot. Put it over high heat and bring to a boil.

Reduce heat to medium. Let it simmer for 15 minutes. Add parsley and basil to the soup.

Fresh Vegetable Soup

Prep Time	:	35 minutes
Cook Time	:	15 minutes
Smart Points per serving	:	0
1 Serving	:	1 cup

This recipe is good for 12 servings.

You will need:

- 2 cloves garlic, minced
- 2 medium carrots, diced
- 2 cups cauliflower, cut into florets
- 2 cups cabbage, shredded
- 2 tsp fresh thyme, coarsely chopped
- 2 cups Swiss chard, chopped
- 1 rib medium celery, coarsely chopped
- 2 cups broccoli, cut into florets
- 1 medium onion, diced
- 2 small zucchinis, diced
- 1 medium sweet red pepper, diced
- 6 cups reduced sodium vegetable broth
- 2 tbsps. fresh lemon juice
- 2 tbsps. fresh parsley, chopped
- 1/2 tsp salt
- 1/4 tsp black pepper

How to do it:

Prepare a large soup pot and put all the ingredients, except parsley and lemon juice. Cover the pot and put it over high heat. Bring it to a boil.

Reduce heat to low and let it simmer for 10 minutes. Uncover the pot and stir in lemon juice and parsley. Add salt and pepper to taste.

Beef, Mushroom, and Barley Soup

Prep Time	:	14 minutes
Cook Time	:	70 minutes
Smart Points per serving	:	6
1 Serving	:	2 cups

This recipe is good for 6 servings.

You will need:

- 16oz lean beef round, cut into 1-inch cubes
- 3 medium carrots, diced
- 2 medium onions, finely chopped
- 3 ribs medium celery, chopped
- 3/4 cup pearl barley
- 1 1/2 cups lima beans, cooked
- 1 1/2 cup cremini mushrooms, sliced
- 7 cups water
- 1 1/2 tsp salt
- 1/4 tsp black pepper

How to do it:

Prepare a large pot with water and put it over high heat. Drop beef and barley. Bring to a boil.

Add carrots, celery, onions, pepper, and salt. Allow the soup to boil for a while. Reduce heat to low and simmer for 45 minutes.

Add in the lima beans and mushrooms. Simmer until the beef is cooked. Serve.

Garden Vegetable Soup

Prep Time	:	20 minutes
Cook Time	:	30 minutes
Smart Points per serving	:	0
1 Serving	:	1 cup

This recipe is good for 6 servings.

You will need:

- 2 cloves garlic, minced
- 1/2 cup carrots, cooked and sliced
- 1/2 tsp dried basil
- 1/4 cup onions, chopped
- 1/2 cup sweet red peppers, diced
- 1/2 cup zucchini, diced
- 3 cups fat-free broth
- 1/2 cup fresh spinach, chopped
- 2 tsp canned tomato paste
- 1/4 tsp dried oregano
- 1/4 tsp salt
- Cooking spray

Procedure:

Spray some oil on a large saucepan and put it over medium heat. Add the onion, garlic, carrot, and pepper. Sauté for a while before you pour in the broth.

Add oregano, cabbage, salt, tomato paste, basil, and spinach. Bring to a boil.

Reduce heat and let it simmer for 15 minutes. Add the zucchini and cook for another 3 or 4 minutes. Serve hot.

Chicken and Root Vegetables Soup

Prep Time	:	15 minutes
Cook Time	:	30 minutes
Smart Points per serving	:	5
1 Serving	:	1/4 of the soup

This recipe is good for 4 servings.

You will need:

- 1 medium carrot, peeled
- 120g parsnip, peeled
- 2 cloves garlic, crushed
- 1 whole leek, trimmed and thinly sliced
- 375g skinless chicken thigh, thinly sliced
- 1 tbsp. fresh parsley, chopped
- 2 tsp olive oil
- 1 medium potato
- 3 cups chicken stock
- 400g tomatoes, diced

How to do it:

Cut the carrot and parsnip into 1cm pieces.

Put a large casserole over medium heat and add some oil. Drop the garlic, leek, carrot, and parsnip. Stir and cook for 5 minutes.

Add tomatoes and stock. Bring it to a boil. Add potato and chicken. Let it simmer for 12 to 15 minutes. Stir in parsley and serve.

Dessert Recipes

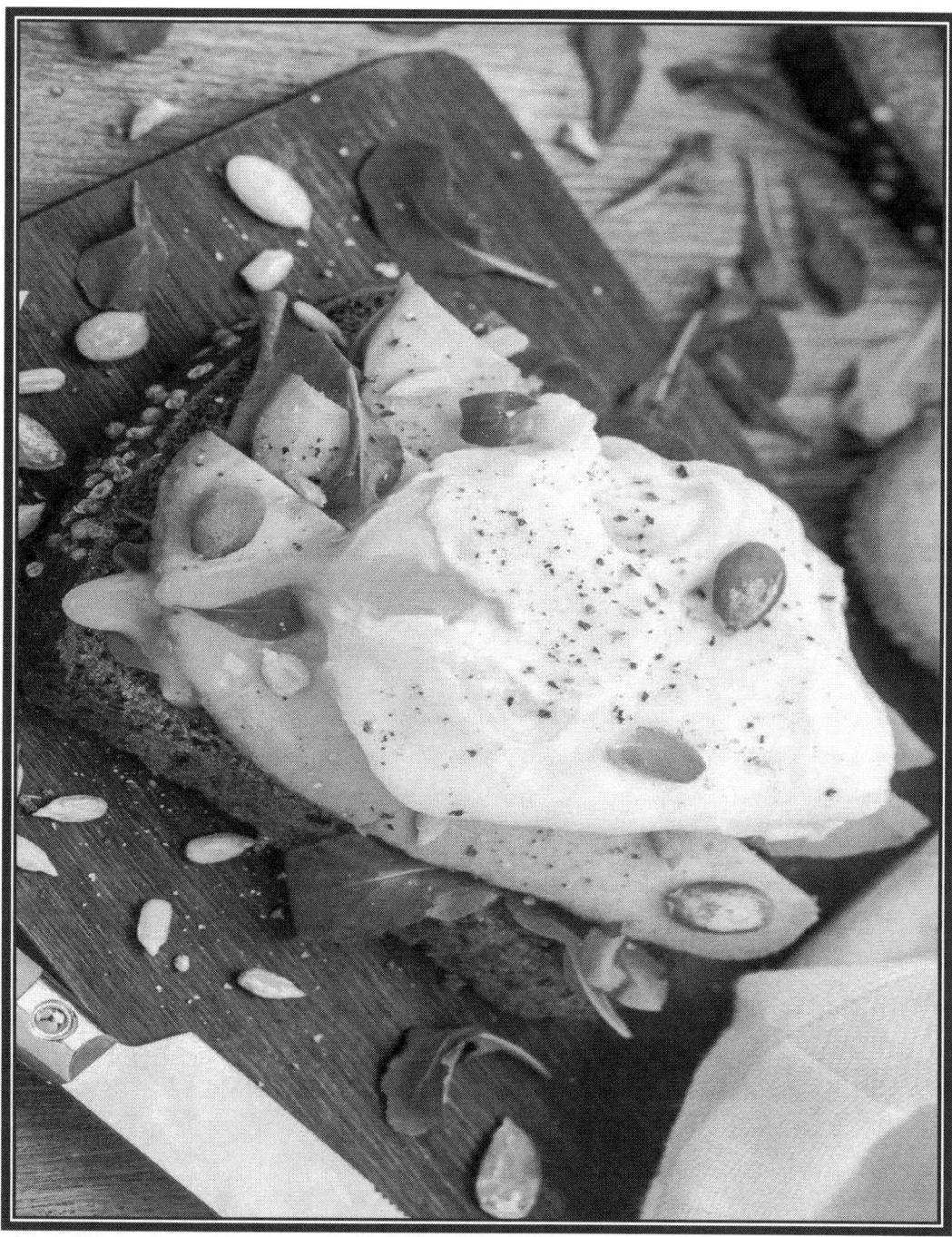

These desserts can take away the blues away.

Ultimate Fruit Salad

Prep Time	:	20 minutes	
Cook Time	:	n/a	
Smart Points per serving	:	4	
1 Serving	:	1/4 of the recipe	

This recipe is good for 4 servings.

You will need:

- 250g fresh strawberries, cut in half
- 300g watermelon, cubed
- 1 tbsp. caster sugar
- 125g fresh blueberries
- 2 medium oranges
- 100g fresh grapes, cut in half
- 200g mango sorbet ice cream stick

How to do it:

Get a large bowl and combine all the fruits, except oranges.

Use a small knife to separate the segments of 1 orange. Squeeze the juice of the other orange. Get a small bowl and mix the orange juice and sugar.

Pour the juice mixture into the salad bowl and add the orange segments. Toss to mix. Cover the bowl and refrigerate for 3 hours or overnight. Divide the fruit salad into 4 equal portions.

Crunchy Chocolate Mousse with Strawberries

Prep Time	:	10minutes
Cook Time	:	n/a
Smart Points per serving	:	4
1 Serving	:	1/4 of the recipe

This recipe is good for 4 servings.

You will need:

- 12 pieces fresh strawberries, chopped
- 100ml skim milk
- 2 pieces chocolate bar, chopped
- 2 packets 20g-chocolate mousse mix

How to do it:

Transfer the milk to a medium bowl. Add in the mousse powder, and use an electric mixer to beat the mixture. Select low speed and gradually increase it until the mixture becomes light and fluffy.

Add two-thirds of strawberry and chocolate bar in the mixture. Fold gently. Divide the mousse mixture into 4 and put each portion in a glass. Refrigerate for 1 hour.

Use the remaining chocolate and strawberry as toppings.

Ricotta and Almond Stuffed Dates

Prep Time	:	5 minutes
Cook Time	:	5 minutes
Smart Points per serving	:	5
1 Serving	:	2 dates

This recipe is good for 4 servings.

You will need:

- 90g low-fat ricotta cheese
- 10ml hazel nut-flavored liqueur
- 45g dark chocolate, melted
- 2 tbsps. almonds, flaked
- 8 pieces fresh dates
- 1 tsp icing sugar

How to do it:

Preheat oven to 350°F. Scatter the almonds on a baking tray and toast in the oven for 3 to 5 minutes. Set aside to cool before you chop them.

Prepare a small baking tray lined with baking paper. Use a small knife to cut the side of each date to remove the seed.

Combine the toasted almonds, icing sugar, ricotta, and liqueur in a bowl. Fill each date with a teaspoon of almond mixture.

Dip half of each date in the melted chocolate. Put the chocolate dipped date on a tray. Do the same with the rest of the dates. Keep them at room temperature for 30 minutes.

Grilled Mango with Raspberry Granita

Prep Time	:	10 minutes
Cook Time	:	5 minutes
Smart Points per serving	:	1
1 Serving	:	2 mango cheeks

This recipe is good for 4 servings.

You will need:

- 4 medium mangoes
- 1 tbsp. icing sugar
- 1 tbsp. fresh mint
- 1/2 cup frozen raspberries
- Some ice cubes

How to do it:

Preheat the grill. Cut off the mango cheeks and leave the seed in the middle. Create a crisscross pattern when slicing the flesh of the mango cheeks – don't cut through the skin. The skin must be intact to hold the flesh. Grill the mango, cut side down, until lightly charred.

Drop the ice cubes, sugar, and raspberries into the food processor. Pulse until the ingredients blended well.

Top each grilled mango cheek with mint and raspberry granita.

Blueberry Pie

Prep Time	:	15 minutes
Cook Time	:	40 minutes
Smart Points per serving	:	7
1 Serving	:	1 slice

This recipe is good for 8 servings.

You will need:

- 375g fresh blueberries
- 4 scoops low-fat ice cream
- 2 tsp sugar
- 1 3/4 reduced-fat short crust pastry, just thawed
- 1 tbsp. corn flour
- 1 tsp fresh lemon rind
- 1 tbsp. caster sugar

How to do it:

Combine the blueberries, corn flour, caster sugar, and lemon rind in a bowl.

Prepare a pie tin with a 22cm diameter and removable base. Place a pastry sheet at the bottom of the pie tin. Cut off the excess pastry. Pour the blueberry mixture into the pie tin with pastry sheet. Spread the mixture evenly.

Slice the rest of the pastry sheet into wide strips. Arrange the strips in a lattice pattern on the pie's top. Trim the strips to fit the pie tin's surface. Press the edges to seal and refrigerate for 30 minutes.

Preheat oven to 350°F. Take out the pie from the fridge. Prepare some water and brush it on the pastry. Sprinkle some sugar. Place the pie tin on a baking tray. Put it in the oven and bake for 40minutes. Let it cool for a bit. Cut into 8 equal slices.

Peaches and Cream Tart

Prep Time	:	15 minutes
Cook Time	:	20 minutes
Smart Points per serving	:	5
1 Serving	:	1 slice

This recipe is good for 10 servings.

How to do it:

- 2 cups peaches in can, sliced
- 100g light cream cheese
- 2 tbsps. almonds, toasted and flaked
- 1 sheet reduced-fat short crust pastry, thawed
- 200g reduced-fat ricotta cheese
- 1 tsp vanilla bean paste
- 1 tbsp. caster sugar
- 1 tsp icing sugar for dusting
- Uncooked rice or beans to serve as weights

How to do it:

Preheat oven to 350°F. Prepare a rectangular baking dish (preferably 35cm x 12cm). Spread the pastry at the bottom of the baking dish. Trim the excess pastry.

On top of the pastry in the baking dish, place a piece of baking paper and allow the paper to hang over the baking dish. Add uncooked rice or beans as weights and bake for 10 minutes. Remove the weights and paper. Bake the pastry for 10 more minutes. Set aside to cool.

Get the electric mixer and beat ricotta, sugar, cream cheese, and vanilla until smooth. Pour the mixture into the cooled pastry. Arrange the peach slices in an overlapping manner.

Spread the toasted almonds on a tray and dust them with some icing sugar. Sprinkle the almonds on the peaches. Divide the finished product into 10 equal slices.

Baby Chocolate Butterfly Cakes

Prep Time	:	30 minutes
Cook Time	:	15 minutes
Smart Points per serving	:	3
1 Serving	:	1 chocolate muffin

This recipe is good for 24 servings.

You will need:

- 100g light cream cheese
- 1 cup white self-rising flour
- 2 tbsps. icing sugar
- 4 tbsps. cocoa powder
- 60g canola spread, melted
- 1/4 cup caster sugar
- 1 medium egg
- 1 tsp icing sugar for dusting
- Oil spray
- 1/2 cup buttermilk

How to do it:

Preheat oven to 350°F. Prepare 2 muffin pans with 12 holes each and can hold 1 1/2 tablespoons of mixture. Put a paper muffin cup that can fit in each hole.

Sift 2 tablespoons cocoa and flour in a large bowl. Stir in caster sugar. Beat egg in a bowl and add buttermilk. Fold the egg mixture into the flour mixture, blend well.

Fill the muffin holes with equal amounts of muffin mixture. Bake for 15 to 20 minutes. Remove the muffin pans from the oven. Let it rest for 5 minutes. Transfer the cooked muffins to a wire rack.

Get an electric mixer and beat the cream cheese in a bowl until smooth. Add the 2 tablespoons icing sugar little by little. Add the remaining cocoa, and beat everything until smooth.

Slice the muffin tops and set aside. Top each muffin with cream cheese mixture. Split the removed muffin top in two and put them on the cream cheese mixture like a pair of butterfly wings. Do the same with the rest. Dust with icing sugar.

Apricot Dessert Quesadillas

Prep Time	:	10 minutes
Cook Time	:	14 minutes
Smart Points per serving	:	3
1 Serving	:	1/2 quesadilla

This recipe is good for 8 servings.

You will need:

- 4 medium whole wheat tortillas
- 4 medium fresh apricots, thinly sliced
- 1 tsp fresh lemon juice
- 1 tbsp. powdered sugar
- 1/2 tsp lemon zest, grated
- 1 tbsp. granulated sugar
- 1/2 cup low-fat cream cheese
- Cooking spray

How to do it:

Combine cream cheese, lemon zest, granulated sugar, and lemon juice in a bowl. Spread the tortilla on a flat surface. Put 1/4 of the mixture on the half of tortilla and top it with 1/4 slice of apricot. Cover it with the other half of tortilla. Do the same with the rest of the tortillas.

Spray some oil on a 12-inch skillet and put over medium heat. Put 2 quesadillas in the skillet. Flip the quesadilla when the bottom side turns golden brown. Cook the other side. Put the cooked quesadillas on a platter. Do the same with the rest of the quesadillas.

Cut each quesadilla in half and sprinkle with powdered sugar.

Spiced Turkish Mocha

Prep Time	:	10 minutes
Cook Time	:	5 minutes
Smart Points per serving	:	4
1 Serving	:	1/4 of the recipe

This recipe is good for 4 servings.

You will need:

- 60g low fat whipped cream
- 600ml hot water
- 1 cardamom pod
- 2 cloves
- 10g instant coffee granules
- 60g hot chocolate drink
- 1 small cinnamon stick

How to do it:

Prepare a pan of hot water and pour in the chocolate drink and coffee granules. Stir in the spices and bring to a simmer.

Turn off the stove and cover the pan. Allow the flavors to infuse for 5 minutes.

Prepare 4 cups and strain the concoction. Discard the spices. Add whipped cream on top of each cup.

Snack Recipes

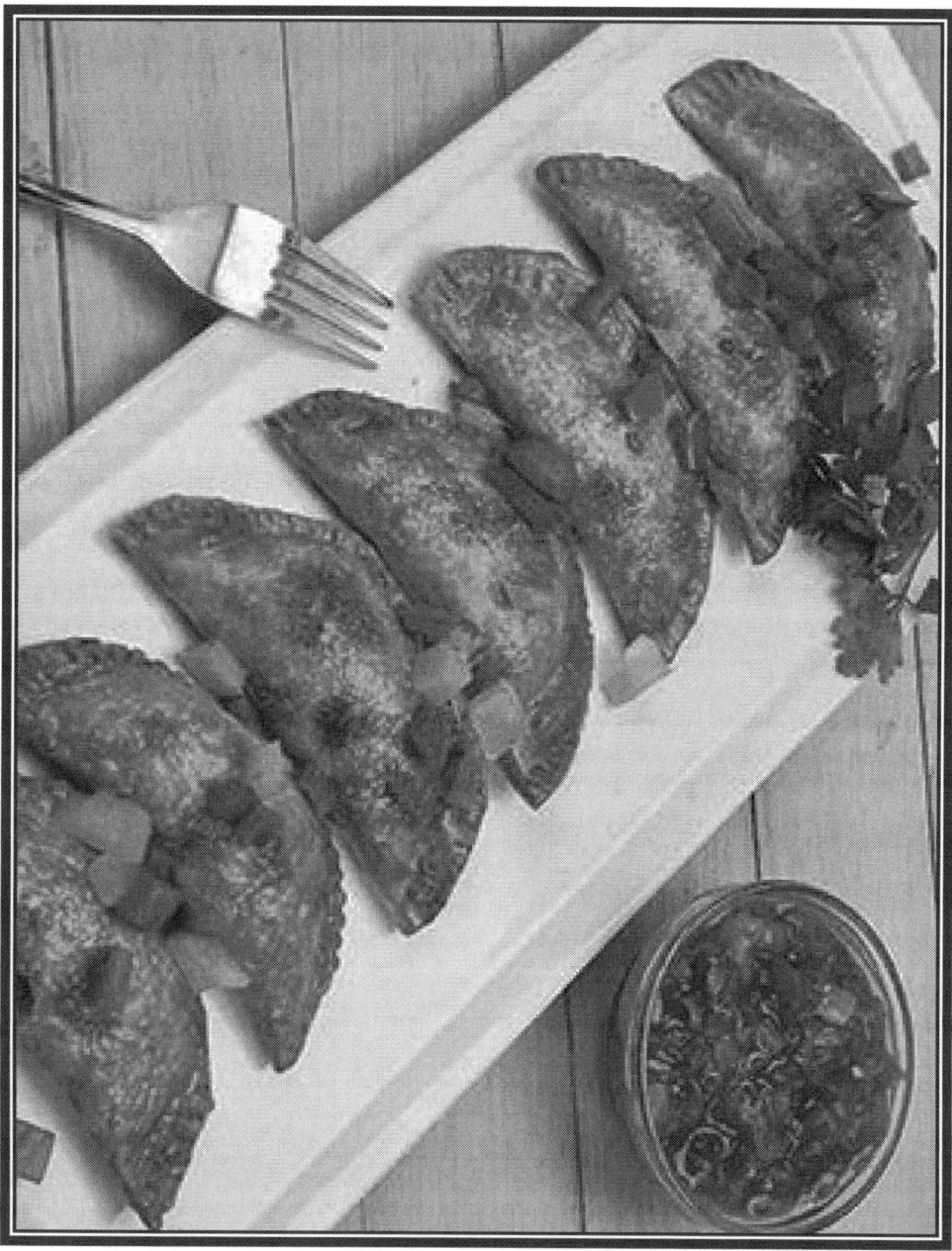

How about some quick snacks to try?

Fruit Salad with Spiced Pistachio Yoghurt

Prep Time	:	15 minutes
Cook Time	:	5 minutes
Smart Points per serving	:	4
1 Serving	:	1/4 of the recipe

This recipe is good for 4 servings.

You will need:

- 1 medium mango, cut into bite-size pieces
- 200g pineapple, peeled and cut into bite-size pieces
- 250g fresh strawberries halved
- 300g Nestle Soleil Vanilla Yoghurt
- 1 tbsp. honey
- 2 medium kiwifruits, peeled and cut into bite-size pieces
- 1/4 cup mint leaves, torn
- 1 medium fresh passion fruit, pulp removed
- 1/2 tsp ground allspice
- 1/4 cup pistachios, toasted and chopped

How to do it:

Put the pineapple, kiwifruit, mint, strawberries, mango, and passion fruit in a large bowl. Mix well and set aside.

Combine half of the toasted pistachios, mixed spice, honey, and yogurt in another bowl. Mix well.

Put a portion of fruit salad in a small bowl with the spiced pistachio yogurt on top.

Sultana and Apple Slice

Prep Time	:	20 minutes
Cook Time	:	20 minutes
Smart Points per serving	:	3
1 Serving	:	1 slice

This recipe is good for 24 servings.

You will need:

- 2 large apples, coarsely grated
- 25g desiccated coconut, grated
- 1 cup self-rising flour
- 150g Nestle Soleil Vanilla Yoghurt
- 1/4 tsp baking soda
- 3/4 cup icing sugar
- 1 medium egg
- 1/4 cup brown sugar
- 5g canola spread
- 1/4 cup sultanas
- 1 tbsp. lemon juice

How to do it:

Preheat oven to 350°F. Spray some oil on a 20cm x 30cm baking dish. Put baking paper on the sides and bottom of the baking dish.

Beat the egg and yogurt in a bowl. Mix well. Stir in apple.

Sift flour and baking soda together in a bowl to blend well. Add sultanas and brown, and mix well to combine. Poke the center of the flour mixture to create a small well and pour in the yogurt mixture. Combine everything thoroughly.

Transfer the mixture to the baking dish and bake for 25 minutes.

Put the icing sugar in a bowl. Add lemon juice and canola spread. Blend until thoroughly combined. Spread the icing on top of the cooked sultana and apple. Sprinkle the coconut on top. Cut into 24 squares and serve.

Strawberry and Blueberry Muffins

Prep Time	:	10 minutes
Cook Time	:	20 minutes
Smart Points per serving	:	4
1 Serving	:	1 muffin

This recipe is good for 12 servings.

You will need:

- 125g fresh blueberries
- 1/4 cup caster sugar
- 1 1/4 cups skim milk
- 1/4 cup dried strawberries
- 1/2 cup strawberry diet jam
- 2 tsp lemon rind
- 2 cups white self-rising flour, sifted
- 1 small egg, lightly beaten
- Cooking spray

How to do it:

Preheat oven to 350°F. Prepare a 12-hole muffin pan and coat each hole with oil spray.

Mix sugar and flour in a large bowl. Combine egg, milk, and rind in another bowl. Add in the blueberries. Make sure to blend everything well.

Add the milk and blueberries mixture to the flour mixture. Whisk everything well.

Fill half of each muffin hole with the mixture. Add 2 tsp of strawberry jam in the center of each muffin mixture. Top each muffin hole with the remaining mixture. Put two slices of dried strawberry on top.

Bake for 18 to 20 minutes. Let cool and serve.

Berry Bliss Balls

Prep Time	:	5 minutes
Cook Time	:	n/a
Smart Points per serving	:	2
1 Serving	:	1 Berry Bliss Ball

This recipe is good for 25 servings.

You will need:

- 150g dried mixed berries
- 3/4 cup wheat germ
- 75g non-fat vanilla yogurt, artificially sweetened
- 1/2 cup raw almonds, finely chopped
- 1/2 cup rolled oats
- 70g dried blueberries

How to do it:

Put the berry mix and blueberries in a bowl. Pour boiling water in a bowl. Soak the berries for 5 minutes to soften. Drain the water and set the berries aside.

Get a food processor and drop in the berries and yogurt. Blend until smooth. Add the wheat germs and oats. Continue blending. When you get a smooth consistency, pour it into a bowl. Cover the bowl and refrigerate the mixture for an hour.

Divide the mixture into 25 equal parts. Roll each part into a ball. Spread the almonds on a plate. Coat each ball with chopped almonds. You can store the balls in an airtight jar and you can keep it in the fridge for five days.

Cauliflower, Mint, and Feta Fritters

Prep Time	:	10 minutes
Cook Time	:	30 minutes
Smart Points per serving	:	1
1 Serving	:	1 fritter

This recipe is good for 6 servings.

You will need:

- 1/4 cup self-rising flour
- 2 tbsps. mint leaves, finely chopped
- 300g cauliflower, cut into florets
- 1 medium egg, lightly beaten
- 20g feta cheese, crumbled
- Cooking spray

How to do it:

Put the cauliflower florets in a steamer and steam until tender. Drain and set aside. Prepare your food processor and blend the cooked florets until you achieve a smooth consistency. Transfer it to a bowl. Stir in feta, flour, egg, and mint. Combine well and season with salt and pepper.

Put some oil in a frying pan over medium heat. Drop the cauliflower batter by tablespoonful into the pan. Cook each side of the fritter until golden brown.

Bacon Bundled Asparagus

Prep Time	:	8 minutes
Cook Time	:	18 minutes
Smart Points per serving	:	2
1 Serving	:	1 bundle

This recipe is good for 4 servings.

You will need:

- 4 slices turkey bacon
- 12 spears of asparagus with uniform thickness, tough ends removed
- Cooking spray

How to do it:

Preheat oven to 400°F. Get 4 asparagus spears and spiral-wrap a slice of bacon around them. Do the same with the rest.

Get a baking sheet and coat it with cooking spray. Put each asparagus with bacon wrapping in the baking dish. Bake for about 18 minutes. Don't forget to flip each bundle halfway through.

Spicy Popcorn

Prep Time		:	5 minutes
Cook Time		:	5 minutes
Smart Points per serving		:	4
1 Serving		:	1/4 of the recipe

This recipe is good for 4 servings.

You will need:

- 60g popcorn kernels
- 1 tbsp. canola oil
- 2 tsp garlic powder
- 1/2 tsp chili flakes
- 2 tsp dried oregano
- 1 tsp lime rind, grated
- 2 tsp dried parsley
- 2 tsp Moroccan seasoning
- 1/2 tsp chili flakes
- 2 tsp dried coriander
- 2 tsp lemon pepper seasoning
- 1 tsp fresh lemon rind, grated
- 1 tsp sea salt, Moroccan spice
- 1 tsp sea salt

How to do it:

Leave the popcorn and canola oil behind and put all the ingredients in a large mortar and pestle – you have an option to do it in batches. Pound the ingredients until they come together. Put it in a large bowl with lid.

Put a large lidded saucepan over medium heat and add some oil. When the oil is hot enough, add the popcorn kernels. Let the kernels pop while shaking the covered saucepan over medium heat. You can stop shaking the saucepan when there's no more popping sound, but be careful not to burn the popcorn.

Remove the unpopped kernels and add the popcorn to the spice mixture. Close the lid of the bowl and shake to coat the popcorn with the spicy mixture.

Coconut and Date Muesli Bars

Prep Time	:	20 minutes
Cook Time	:	10 minutes
Smart Points per serving	:	4
1 Serving	:	1 bar

This recipe is good for 24 servings.

You will need:

- 10 pieces fresh dates, pitted and chopped
- 60g desiccated coconut
- 1/2 cup brown sugar
- 3/4 cup wholemeal flour
- 250g dry rolled oats
- 1/4 cup flaxseeds
- 1 tsp baking soda
- 150g Nestle Soleil Vanilla Yoghurt
- 2 medium eggs
- 1/2 cup wheat germ
- Cooking spray

How to do it:

Preheat oven to 350°F. Coat a glass baking dish with oil. Put baking paper on the sides and bottom.

Combine yogurt, egg, and sugar in a saucepan. Stir in dates and continue mixing. Put the flour, baking soda, and wheat germ in a separate bowl.

Combine the flour and yogurt mixture together and blend well. Add coconut, flaxseeds, and oats. Mix until combined.

Get your prepared baking dish and pour in the mixture. Even out the surface. Bake in the oven. Insert a toothpick to see if the inside is already cooked. When the toothpick comes out clean, it is done. Set aside to cool and then cut into 24 bars.

Pepper and Mushroom Kebabs with Dip

Prep Time	:	15 minutes
Cook Time	:	10 minutes
Smart Points per serving	:	0
1 Serving	:	1 kebab + 1 1/2 tbsp. dip

This recipe is good for 8 servings.

You will need:

- 3 medium sweet red peppers, diced
- 16 small cremini mushrooms, cleaned and trimmed
- 1/4 tsp salt
- 1/4 tsp black pepper
- Cooking spray

Things you will need for the dip:

- 1 clove garlic, minced
- 1 pinch salt
- 1 tsp dill, chopped
- 1/4 cup fat-free sour cream
- 1/2 cup fat-free plain Greek yogurt

How to do it:

Preheat grill to high.

Prepare 8 pieces 12-inch metal skewers. Put 2 mushrooms and 3 pieces of pepper to each skewer. Season the kebabs with salt and pepper and coat each one with cooking spray. Grill each side for about 5 minutes.

To prepare the dip: get a bowl and combine all the ingredients for the dip. Set aside.

Serve each kebab together with dip.

Lemon-Rosemary White Bean Bruschetta

Prep Time	: 18 minutes
Cook Time	: 10 minutes
Smart Points per serving	: 1
1 Serving	: 1 bruschetta

This recipe is good for 30 servings.

You will need:

- 15oz cannellini beans in can, rinsed and drained
- 10oz French baguette bread, cut into 30 slices
- 1/2 tsp lemon zest
- 1 tsp garlic salt
- 2 medium red onions, chopped
- 1 tbsp. olive oil, extra virgin
- 4 medium plum tomatoes, chopped
- 4 tsp fresh lemon juice
- 2 tbsps. grated Parmesan cheese
- 1 tbsp. fresh rosemary, chopped
- 1/4 tsp black pepper, freshly ground
- 1 tsp kosher salt
- Cooking spray

How to do it:

Preheat oven to 375°F. Prepare a baking sheet and line it with foil.

Arrange the bread slices on the baking sheet. Gently coat each side of the bread with cooking spray. Put some garlic salt on top of each slice. Bake for about 5 to 10 minutes.

Get a bowl and combine the remaining ingredients, but leave the lemon zest and cheese behind. Mash the beans using a fork.

Spread a tablespoonful of bean mixture on each slice of bread. Add zest and cheese on top.

Buffalo-Style Stuffed Celery

Prep Time	:	10 minutes
Cook Time	:	n/a
Smart Points per serving	:	1
1 Serving	:	2 pieces

This recipe is good for 10 servings.

You will need:

- 5 ribs of large celery, cut each rib into 4 equal pieces
- 2 1/2 tsp hot pepper sauce
- 1/2 tsp garlic, minced
- 2 tbsps. blue cheese, softened
- 1/2 cup low-fat cream cheese, softened
- 1/4 tsp salt

How to do it:

Combine garlic, blue cheese, salt, and cream cheese in a bowl until smooth. Spread 1/2 tablespoon mixture on each celery piece.

Arrange the stuffed celery on a serving platter, and drizzle each piece with 1/4 teaspoon hot pepper sauce.

Butternut Squash Fries

Prep Time	:	10 minutes
Cook Time	:	18 minutes
Smart Points per serving	:	0
1 Serving	:	4 pieces

This recipe is good for 4 servings.

You will need:

- 1 pound butternut squash, cut into 16 sticks with 3/4 inch thickness
- 1 tsp salt
- Cooking spray

How to do it:

Preheat oven to 450ºF. Coat the baking sheet with some cooking spray.

Scatter the squash sticks on the baking sheet. Season the sticks with salt and lightly coat with cooking spray.

Roast in the oven to turn crispy. Don't forget to flip the fries.

Chocolate-Banana Mini Muffins

Prep Time	:	20 minutes
Cook Time	:	18 minutes
Smart Points per serving	:	2
1 Serving	:	1 muffin

This recipe is good for 36 servings.

You will need:

- 1 large banana, mashed
- 1/2 cup quick oats
- 1/2 tsp baking soda
- 1 cup light vanilla yogurt, artificially sweetened
- 1 1/4 cups all-purpose flour
- 2 tsp baking powder
- 1 whole egg, beaten
- 1/2 cup mini chocolate chips
- 1/2 tsp extract, vanilla
- 1/4 cup unpacked brown sugar
- 1/2 tsp table salt

How to do it:

Preheat oven to 375ºF. Prepare 3 muffin pans with 12 small holes each. Lightly brush or spray each hole with oil.

In a large mixing bowl, whisk together egg, oats, yogurt, milk, and vanilla extract. Let it sit for 5 minutes to soften the oats. Add the mashed banana.

Get another bowl and combine flour, baking powder, brown sugar, baking soda, and salt. Fold the egg mixture gently into the flour mixture. Avoid beating the dough because it will get thick. Set aside 1 tablespoon chocolate chips for later. Add the remaining chocolate chips to the mixture.

Fill each muffin hole with a tablespoon of mixture. Get the tablespoon of chocolate chips and sprinkle some over each muffin. Put the muffins in the oven to bake. To test if the muffins are done, insert a wooden toothpick in the center. The muffins are done when the stick comes out clean.

Roasted Cauliflower with Lemon and Garlic

Prep Time	:	12 minutes
Cook Time	:	30 minutes
Smart Points per serving	:	1
1 Serving	:	2/3 cup

This recipe is good for 8 servings.

You will need:

- 2 medium-sized heads cauliflower, cut into florets
- 1 tbsp. olive oil
- 1 tsp garlic, minced
- 1 1/2 tsp lemon zest
- 1 1/2 tbsps. fresh parsley, chopped
- 1 tsp kosher salt

How to do it:

Preheat oven to 450ºF. Prepare two large baking sheets and coat them with cooking spray.

Put the florets in a colander, rinse, and drain to dry. Place the florets in a large bowl. Sprinkle some salt and toss. Drizzle oil over the florets.

Scatter the florets evenly on the baking sheets. Put in the oven to roast for 30 minutes. Flip the florets halfway through and continue baking. Place the roasted florets in a large pot. Add lemon zest, parsley, and garlic. Toss to coat the florets evenly.

Maple Granola Bars

Prep Time	:	10 minutes
Cook Time	:	30 minutes
Smart Points per serving	:	9
1 Serving	:	1 log

This recipe is good for 10 servings.

You will need:

- 3 cups quick cooking rolled oats
- 1 tbsp. dark brown sugar, packed
- 1/4 cup maple syrup
- 1/4 cup honey
- 1 tsp cinnamon, ground
- 1 cup raisins, chopped
- 1/4 cup water
- 1/2 cup almonds, chopped
- 1/2 tsp salt

How to do it:

Preheat the oven to 325°F. Squirt some nonstick spray on the baking sheet.

Get a large bowl and combine almonds, oats, raisins, cinnamon, and salt.

Pour water in a saucepan and add syrup, honey, and brown sugar. Place it over medium heat and bring the mixture to a boil. Turn off the stove and pour the syrup into the almond mixture. Blend well.

Divide the mixture into 10 equal portions. Wet your hands and shape each portion of mixture into a 4-inch long log. Arrange the logs on the baking sheet and press each one to achieve half inch thickness.

Put the tray in the oven and bake for about 30 minutes. Allow it to cool.

Slow Cook Recipes

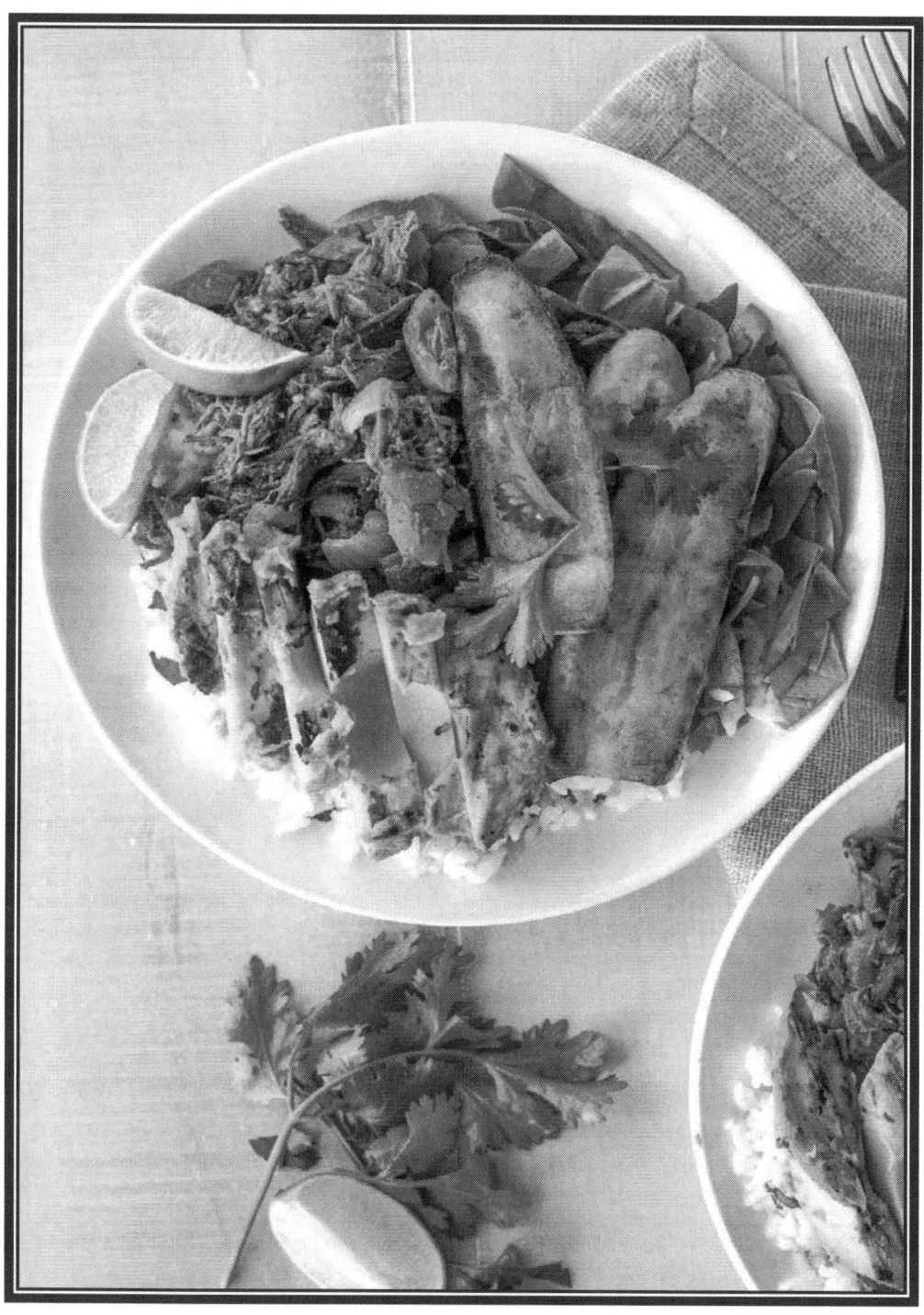

Crock Pot Loaded Beef Stew:

Serving Size: 1 cup
Servings per Recipe: 8
Smart Points per Serving: 8
Calories: 274
Cooking Time: 8 Hours

Ingredients:

1. 2 tablespoons olive oil
2. 1 pound lean hamburger stew meat, cubed in around 1-inch pieces
3. 2 tablespoons flour for covering the hamburger
4. 1 cup red wine, (discretionary non-alcoholic wine or vegetable juices)
5. 5 red potatoes, cubed
6. 1 white onion, diced
7. 1 cup carrots, sliced/cubed
8. 1 cup celery, sliced/cubed
9. 1/2 cup mushrooms cut
10. 1 cup peas, frozen or fresh
11. 4 garlic cloves, minced
12. 1/4 cup tomato puree
13. 1 tablespoon soy sauce
14. 2 tablespoons horseradish
15. 2 cups low sodium hamburger juices
16. 3 tablespoons balsamic vinegar
17. 2 narrows bay leaves
18. 2 sprigs fresh thymes
19. 1 teaspoon dried parsley
20. 1 teaspoon dried oregano
21. 1 teaspoon black pepper
22. 1/2 teaspoon sea salt

Nutrition Information:

1. Saturated Fat: 2g
2. Cholesterol: 37mg
3. Sodium: 532mg
4. Carbohydrates: 37g
5. Fiber: 5g
6. Sugar: 7g
7. Protein: 19g

Directions:

1. Start by heating oil in a skillet over medium-high temperature.
2. Toss the meat in the flour then add to the cooker.
3. Make them brown on all sides for around two minutes—meat doesn't need to be cooked through, simply get a pleasant covering on it!

4. Add wine and blend it to relax the bits off the base of the dish. Bring down warmth to medium and stew for 5 minutes.
5. Include the meat, container sauce, and all the rest of the ingredients to the slow cooker. Cover and cook on low for 7 to 8 hours, or high for 4 to 5 hours. Expel the inlet leaves and thyme, and serve!

Thai Chicken Soup:

Serving Size: 1 cup
Servings per Recipe: 8
Smart Points per Serving: 11
Calories: 269
Cooking Time: 4 to 8 Hours

Ingredients:
1. 5 chicken thighs, skinless and boneless
2. 6 cups chicken stock, no fat
3. 1 (14.5 ounces) can coconut milk (full-fat)
4. 1 teaspoon kosher salt
5. 1/2 teaspoon black pepper
6. 4 teaspoons ground ginger
7. 1 teaspoon red curry powder
8. 1 (4.5 ounces) can diced jalapeños
9. 1 red bell pepper, seeded and diced
10. 1 onion, diced
11. 3 carrots, sliced
12. 1 big potato, cut into little shapes
13. Juice of 1 lime
14. 1/4 cup crisply chopped cilantro

Nutrition Information:
1. Saturated Fat: 11g
2. Cholesterol: 25mg
3. Sodium: 812mg
4. Carbohydrates: 24g
5. Fiber: 4g
6. Sugar: 6g
7. Protein: 14g

Directions:
1. Include all ingredients, aside from cilantro, to the slow cooker. Cover and cook on low 6 to 8 hours or high 3 to 4 hours.
2. At the point when carrots are delicate and chicken is done, expel chicken and shred with a fork. Return destroyed chicken and a large portion of the cilantro to the soup. Mix soup and serve!
3. Decorate singular servings with the rest of the cilantro and serve.

Tasty Bourbon Chicken:

Serving Size: 1 cup
Servings per Recipe: 5
Smart Points per Serving: 8
Calories: 380
Cooking Time: 4 to 8 Hours

Ingredients:
1. 3 tablespoons molasses or nectar
2. 1/4 cup ketchup
3. 3 tablespoons apple juice vinegar
4. 1/4 cup water
5. 5 boneless skinless chicken breasts
6. 1/2 teaspoon ground ginger
7. 4 cloves garlic, minced
8. 1/4 teaspoon pounded red stew drops
9. 1/4 cup sans sugar squeezed apple
10. 1/4 cup (great quality) Bourbon
11. 1/4 cup low-sodium soy sauce
12. 1 teaspoon Kosher or sea salt
13. 1/2 teaspoon black pepper
14. 1/4 cup cut green onions, decorate

Nutrition Information:
1. Saturated Fat: 1g
2. Cholesterol: 172mg
3. Sodium: 745mg
4. Carbohydrates: 17g
5. Fiber: 0g
6. Sugar: 14g
7. Protein: 32g

Directions:
1. Put chicken breasts into a moderate cooker.
2. Whisk together all the rest of the ingredients in a bowl then pour over chicken. Cook on low 4-5 hours or high for 2-3 hours.
3. When cooking is finished, evacuate chicken and shred it.
4. Return chicken to moderate cooker and cook on low for an additional 15 minutes.
5. On the off chance that coveted, serve over cocoa rice with green onions on top.

Protein Chicken Tacos:

Serving Size: 1
Servings per Recipe: 8
Smart Points per Serving: 11
Calories: 382
Cooking Time: 4 to 8 Hours

Ingredients:
1. 1 pound boneless skinless chicken breast
2. 3 cups no sugar included salsa
3. 1 teaspoon ground cumin
4. 2 tablespoons stew powder
5. 1/2 cup corn kernels
6. 1/2 cup black beans
7. 1/2 cup low sodium chicken soup
8. 8 entire wheat flour tortillas
9. 1 cup destroyed Romaine lettuce
10. 1 huge tomato, diced
11. 1 cup low-fat grated cheddar
12. 1/4 cup diced avocado
13. 1/4 cup plain Greek yogurt

Nutrition Information:
1. Saturated Fat: 4g
2. Cholesterol: 57mg
3. Sodium: 1237mg
4. Carbohydrates: 44g
5. Fiber: 6g
6. Sugar: 7g
7. Protein: 26g

Directions:
1. In a slow cooker, include chicken, salsa, cumin, black beans, chili powder, corn, and juices.
2. Cook on low for 8 hours or high for 4 hours. Remove delicate chicken from cooker and shred with a fork. Come back to a moderate cooker and cook for an additional 30 minutes on low or 15 minutes on high.
3. Spoon around 2 tablespoons of destroyed chicken into every tortilla. Beat with lettuce, tomato, cheddar, avocado, and yogurt. Serve and appreciate!

Sweet Potato Chili:

Serving Size: 1 cup
Servings per Recipe: 6 cup
Smart Points per Serving: 8
Calories: 275
Cooking Time: 6 to 8 Hours
Ingredients:

1. 1 pound ground turkey
2. 1 sweet onion, diced
3. 1 jalapeno, seeded and minced
4. 3 garlic cloves, minced
5. 2 sweet potatoes, cubed
6. 1 (14.5 ounces) can dark beans
7. 1 (14.5 ounces) fire simmered pulverized tomatoes
8. 2 cups low-sodium chicken juices
9. 1 teaspoon cinnamon
10. 1 tablespoon bean stew powder
11. 1 teaspoon cumin
12. 1 teaspoon sea salt
13. 1/2 teaspoon dark pepper
14. 1 tablespoon unsweetened cocoa powder

Nutrition Information:

1. Saturated Fat: 2g
2. Cholesterol: 52mg
3. Sodium: 676mg
4. Carbohydrates: 33g
5. Fiber: 9g
6. Sugar: 8g
7. Protein: 23g

Directions:

1. Add all ingredients to the slow cooker, separating the ground turkey into bits with a wood spoon. Blend to consolidate. Boil on low flame for 6 to 8 hours or high flame for 3 to 4 hours.
2. On the off chance that coveted, present with a dab of sour cream or Greek yogurt and entire grain tortillas disintegrated on top.

One Pot Pumpkin Chili:

Serving Size: 1 cup
Servings per Recipe: 6 cup
Smart Points per Serving: 7
Calories: 214
Cooking Time: 6 to 8 Hours

Ingredients:
1. 1 onion, diced
2. 2 (14 ounce) cans crushed tomatoes
3. 2 (14 ounces) cans black beans, a drained
4. 1 carrot, shredded
5. 1 bell pepper, diced
6. 1 jalapeno, veins and seeds removed and minced
7. 2 cloves garlic, minced
8. 1 1/2 cups pumpkin puree
9. 1 cups low sodium vegetable broth
10. 2 tablespoons chili powder
11. 1 teaspoon pumpkin pie spice
12. 1 teaspoon kosher salt
13. 1/2 teaspoon black pepper

Nutrition Information:
1. Saturated Fat: 0g
2. Cholesterol: 0mg
3. Sodium: 841mg
4. Carbohydrates: 43g
5. Fiber: 16g
6. Sugar: 11g
7. Protein: 12g

Directions:
Add everything to your slow cooker and stir to combine. Cook on low for 5 to 6 hours or high for 2 to 3 hours. Present with a spoonful of Greek yogurt or avocado slices.

Apple Butter Pulled Pork:

Serving Size: 1 cup
Servings per Recipe: 6 cup
Smart Points per Serving: 12
Calories: 352
Cooking Time: 2 Hours
Ingredients:

1. 5 apples, peeled, cored and diced
2. 2 teaspoons cinnamon
3. 1/2 teaspoon nutmeg
4. 1/4 teaspoon allspice
5. 1/4 teaspoon ground cloves
6. 1/4 cup coconut sugar
7. 1/4 cup apple cider vinegar
8. 3 cloves of garlic, minced
9. 1 medium onion, chopped
10. 1 tablespoon spicy brown mustard
11. 1 teaspoon kosher salt
12. 1/2 teaspoon black pepper
13. 4 pork loin chops

Nutrition Information:

1. Saturated Fat: 4g
2. Cholesterol: 92mg
3. Sodium: 426mg
4. Carbohydrates: 33g
5. Fiber: 5g
6. Sugar: 23g
7. Protein: 28g

Directions:

1. Place apples, cinnamon, nutmeg, allspice and coconut sugar into slow cooker. Cook on low for four hours, or high for two hours.
2. Add cider vinegar, garlic, onion, mustard, salt, and pepper. Combine the apples (they should be mushy enough that you can mash them), then adjoin pork chops. Wrap the chops with the apple mix. Cook for an additional four hours on low down temperature, or maximum two hours on high flame. Remove pork, shred and return to the slow cooker. Roast on high flame for ten more minutes or so, and then serve!

Bean and Potato Soup:

Serving Size: 1 1/2 cup
Servings per Recipe: 8 cup
Smart Points per Serving: 8
Calories: 287
Cooking Time: 8 Hours

Ingredients:
1. 1 pound Yukon gold potatoes, peeled and slashed (around 3-4 cups crushed)
2. 2 jars northern beans, drained and cleansed
3. 1/2 cup slashed onions or shallots
4. 2 garlic cloves, minced
5. 1/2 cup slashed carrots
6. 1/2 cup slashed celery
7. 2 tablespoons finely slashed new rosemary or 2 teaspoons dried rosemary
8. 1/2 tablespoon finely slashed new oregano or 1 teaspoon dried oregano
9. 2 tablespoons crisp thyme leaves or 2 teaspoons dried thyme
10. 1 teaspoon fit or ocean salt
11. 1/4 teaspoon dark pepper
12. 1 teaspoon pounded red pepper chips, discretionary, pretty much for heat fancied
13. 4 cups low-sodium vegetable or chicken stock
14. 1 parmesan skin or 1 (2-inch) piece parmesan, optional*
15. 1 tablespoon additional virgin olive oil
16. 1 bay leaf

Nutrition Information:
1. Saturated Fat: 1g
2. Cholesterol: 2mg
3. Sodium: 91mg
4. Carbohydrates: 53g
5. Fiber: 10g
6. Sugars: 2g
7. Protein: 13g

Directions:
1. Add all fixings to the simmering pot and mix. Permit to cook on low for 6-8 hours or high for 5 hours.
2. *Note that including the parmesan skin or a bit of parmesan includes a considerable measure of appetizing flavor to the soup. Expel it before serving.

White Bean and Chicken Chili:

Serving Size: 1 cup
Servings per Recipe: 12 cup
Smart Points per Serving: 8
Calories: 315
Cooking Time: 8 Hours

Ingredients:

1. 2 pounds boneless, skinless chicken breasts, cut into bite on pieces (around 1/2-inch)
2. 1 little sweet onion, diced
3. 2 cloves garlic, minced
4. 2 jalapeño peppers, seeded and diced
5. 1 medium Poblano pepper, seeded and diced
6. 2 (4 ounces) jars diced green chilies
7. 1 teaspoon legitimate or ocean salt, pretty much to taste
8. 1 tablespoon stew powder
9. 2 teaspoons cumin
10. 1/2 teaspoon black pepper
11. 1 teaspoon dried oregano
12. 1/4 cup newly cleaved cilantro
13. 3 (15-ounce) jars cannellini beans (discretionary naval force beans), depleted
14. 4 cups chicken soup, sans fat, low-sodium
15. 1/2 cup decreased fat ground cheddar
16. 1 cup low-fat sour cream or Greek yogurt

Nutrition Information:

1. Saturated Fat: 3g
2. Cholesterol: 69mg
3. Sodium: 223mg
4. Carbohydrates: 31g
5. Fiber: 6g
6. Sugars: 4g
7. Protein: 30g

Directions:

1. Include all ingredients, with the exception of cheddar and yogurt, to the moderate cooker, blend to join, wrap and cook on low temperature for 6-8 hours or high temperature for 3-4 hours. The most recent 30 minutes of cooking time, include the harsh cream and cheddar, blend to consolidate. Cover and keep cooking 30 minutes.
2. On the off chance that covered, before serving orderly with sour cream, cheddar, and cilantro.

Chicken and Rice Casserole:

Serving Size: 1 cup
Servings per Recipe: 4
Smart Points per Serving: 9
Calories: 327
Cooking Time: 8 Hours

Ingredients:
1. 4 (1.5 pounds) new boneless, skinless chicken thighs or bosoms, cut into pieces of around 1-inch
2. 1 tablespoon additional virgin olive oil
3. 3 cups chicken stock, no fat
4. 2 vast carrots, peeled and cut into 1/2-inch rounds
5. 1/2 teaspoon fit or sea salt, pretty much to taste
6. 1/4 teaspoon dark pepper
7. 2 cups cooked cocoa rice or quinoa
8. 1 cup (defrosted) peas
9. 1/2 cup ground parmesan cheddar

Nutrition Information:
1. Saturated Fat: 3 g
2. Sodium: 833 mg
3. Cholesterol: 78 mg
4. Carbohydrates: 36 g
5. Fiber: 3 g
6. Sugars: 6 g
7. Protein: 25 g

Directions:
1. In the slow cooker, include the chicken, olive oil, carrots, juices, salt, and pepper. Cover up and cook on low temperature for 6 to 8 hours or on high flame for 3 to 4, or until chicken is done and carrots delicate.
2. Whenever cooked, include pre-cooked rice, peas, and parmesan. Blend to join and keep cooking for 10 minutes.

Honey Mustard Chicken:

Serving Size: 1 cup
Servings per Recipe: 4
Smart Points per Serving: 9
Calories: 327
Cooking Time: 8 Hours

Ingredients:

1. 4 (1.5 pounds) new boneless, skinless chicken thighs or breasts, cut into chunks of around 1-inch
2. 1 tablespoon extra-virgin olive oil
3. 3 cups chicken stock, no fat
4. 2 substantial carrots, peeled and cut into 1/2-inch rounds
5. 1/2 teaspoon genuine or ocean salt, pretty much to taste
6. 1/4 teaspoon black pepper
7. 2 cups cooked brown rice or quinoa
8. 1 cup (defrosted) peas
9. 1/2 cup ground parmesan cheddar

Nutrition Information:

1. Saturated Fat: 2 g
2. Sodium: 525 mg
3. Cholesterol: 66 mg
4. Carbohydrates: 19 g
5. Fiber: 1 g
6. Sugars: 17 g
7. Protein: 14 g

Directions:

1. In the cooker, include the chicken, olive oil, carrots, stock, salt, and pepper. Cover up and cook on low temperature for 6 to 8 hours or on high flame for 3 to 4, or until chicken is done and carrots delicate.
2. Whenever cooked, include pre-cooked rice, peas, and parmesan. Blend to join and keep cooking for 10 minutes.

Loaded Creamy Corn Chowder:

Serving Size: 1 ½ cup
Servings per Recipe: 6
Smart Points per Serving: 9
Calories: 269
Cooking Time: Approx. 4 to 8 Hours
Ingredients:
FOR THE CHOWDER:
1. 4 cups vegetable stock
2. 2 cups almond milk, unsweetened or 2 cups canned coconut milk (creamier outcomes)
3. 2 1/2 tablespoons cornstarch
4. 2 tablespoons olive oil
5. 1 teaspoon garlic powder
6. 1 teaspoon onion powder
7. 3/4 teaspoon salt
8. 1/2 teaspoon pepper
9. 2 cups red potato, diced
10. 1 (16-ounce) bundle solidified corn

FOR THE TOPPINGS:
1. 1/4 cup diced tomato
2. 1/4 cup diced purple onion
3. 1/4 cup daintily cut scallions
4. 1/4 cup decreased fat cheddar

Nutrition Information:
1. Saturated Fat: 4 g
2. Cholesterol: 14 mg
3. Sodium: 152 mg
4. Carbohydrates: 34 g
5. Dietary Fiber: 3 g
6. Sugars: 8 g
7. Protein: 10 g

Directions:
1. In a 3-4 quart moderate cooker, whisk together vegetable stock, almond milk, cornstarch, olive oil, garlic powder, onion powder, salt, and pepper. Mix in potato and corn. Cover up and cook on low temperature for 6 to 7 hours or on high flame for 3 to 4 hours. Serve finished with your most loved fixings.
2. *For creamier outcomes, expel 2-3 cups of the chowder before serving and add them to a blender. Puree on high and after that arrival to the soup, blending. On the other hand, you can embed a hand blender (submersion blender) into the soup and puree until covered surface/level of richness is accomplished.

Chunky Squash & Chicken Stew:

Serving Size: 2 cup
Servings per Recipe: 4
Smart Points per Serving: 8
Calories: 297
Cooking Time: Approx. 4 Hours

Ingredients:

1. 15 ounces (boneless and skinless) chicken bosoms, hacked into nibble estimated pieces
2. Flour, for covering
3. 1/2 teaspoon salt
4. 1/8 teaspoon pepper
5. 2 tablespoons additional virgin olive oil
6. 2 1/2 cups chicken juices
7. 1 medium onion, coarsely slashed
8. 14 ounces squash, diced
9. 1-1/2 cups vegetable juices
10. 3 crisp sage leaves, chopped or torn

Nutrition Information:

1. Saturated Fat: 2 g
2. Cholesterol: 69 mg
3. Sodium: 245 mg
4. Carbohydrates: 21 g
5. Sugars: 5 g
6. Protein: 27 g

Directions:

1. Coat the chicken with flour and shake off the abundance. Over medium warmth, in a pan with additional virgin olive oil, chestnut the chicken then season with salt and pepper. Try not to stuff. Cook in clusters if necessary. Pour 1 cup chicken soup in the pan and cook until the sauce thickens.
2. Exchange the substance of the pan to the moderate cooker. Include a smidgen all the more additional virgin olive oil in the pot then sauté the onions over low - medium warmth for around 5 minutes. Exchange the onions to the moderate cooker. Include the squash, staying chicken stock, and sage in the moderate cooker. Set on low for 4 hours.

Cauliflower Fried Rice:

Serving Size: 2 cups
Servings per Recipe: 4
Smart Points per Serving: 5
Calories: 172
Cooking Time: Approx. 4 to 8 Hours

Ingredients:
1. 2 heads cauliflower
2. 2 tablespoons ginger-garlic puree (or new garlic and ginger root, peeled and minced)
3. 1/2 cup vegetable soup
4. 2 eggs
5. 1 cup solidified vegetable blend
6. 1/2 cup Boars Head turkey ham, diced (discretionary)
7. 1/4 cup green onions, diced
8. 1/4 cup cilantro (discretionary)
9. 2 tablespoons lite (low-sodium) soy sauce or to taste

Nutrition Information:
1. Saturated Fat: 2 g
2. Cholesterol: 92 mg
3. Sodium: 405 mg
4. Carbohydrates: 22 g
5. Sugars: 6 g
6. Protein: 13 g

Directions:
1. Cut the florets off each head of cauliflower. Put the florets in an extensive nourishment processor. Beat until finely disintegrated.
2. In an extensive simmering pot, include cauliflower pieces, ginger garlic puree, and vegetable stock. Cover and cook on high for 2 hours or on low for 3-4 hours.
3. 30 minutes prior to plating, beat the eggs together and mix them in a saucepan. Include eggs, solidified veggies, and diced turkey ham (if craved) to the simmering pot. Permit to cook for 30 minutes more, or until the solidified veggies are warm. Mix in green onions and cilantro. Shower with soy sauce to taste. Serve and enjoy!

The Ultimate 3-Month Meal Plan

Here is your 3-month meal plan to get you started and get you going. The sample meal plans are for those who only need to spend 30 Smart Points per day. You can adjust accordingly. Remember to drink lots of water.

Month 1

DAY 1	
Breakfast	6
2 scrambled eggs with milk and butter	6
Apple	0
Snack	4
1/4 cup almonds	4
Mixed berries	0
Lunch	8
Cream of Broccoli	2
Stir-fry Beef & Broc	3
Baby Choc Butterfly	3
Snack	2
2 servings Roasted Cauliflower w/ Lemon and Garlic	2
Dinner	10
Cider-Glazed Pork Chops	9
Grilled Mango w/ Raspberry Granita	1
Total Smart Points	30

DAY 2	
Breakfast	10
Hash and Eggs	8
1 slice bread	2
Snack	3
Sultana & Apple Slice	3
Lunch	7
Fajita-Stuffed Chicken	4
Super Easy Chicken Noodle Soup	3
Snack	4
Fruit Salad w/ Spiced Pistachio Yogurt	4
Dinner	6
Filet Mignon w/ Red Wine Sauce	6
Total Smart Points	30

DAY 3	
Breakfast	7
Steak and Eggs	5
peach	0
1 slice bread	2
Snack	4
Strawberry and Blueberry Muffin	4
Lunch	8
Grilled Vegetable and Haloumi	7
3oz cooked shrimp	1
Snack	5
Spicy Popcorn	4
Cauliflower, Mint and Feta Fritters	1
Dinner	6
Pulled Pork Special	6
Italian-Inspired Vegetable Soup	0
Total Smart Points	30

DAY 4	
Breakfast	8
1 banana	0
Cheesy and Saucy Egg Sandwich	8
Snack	2
hardboiled egg	2
Lunch	9
Caramelized Onion and Mushroom Lasagna	9
Snack	2
Cream of Broccoli Soup	2
Celery	0

DAY 5	
Breakfast	4
Passion Fruit Soufflé	4
nectarine	0
Snack	3
Bacon Bundled Asparagus	2
2 tbsps. low-fat cheddar cheese (shredded)	1
Lunch	8
Spiced Turkish Mocha	4
California Club Wrap	4
Snack	3
1 tbsp. mayonnaise	3
mixed greens	0

DAY 6	
Breakfast	8
3 slices bacon	5
1 fried egg	3
orange	0
Snack	0
Pepper and Mushroom Kebabs w/ Dip	0
Lunch	6
Feta-Stuffed Chicken Burgers	6
Snack	3
3 servings Buffalo Style Stuffed Celery	3

Dinner	9
Baked Vegetable Tart	9
Total Smart Points	**30**

Dinner	12
Sesame-Ginger Pork Tenderloin	6
1 cup cooked rice (brown)	6
Total Smart Points	**30**

Dinner	13
General Tso's Chicken	8
Peaches and Cream Tart	5
Total Smart Points	**30**

DAY 7	
Breakfast	7
1 English Muffin	4
1oz crumbled feta	3
grapes	0
Snack	4
cantaloupe	0
Coconut and Date Muesli Bar	4
Lunch	8
Eggplant Parmigiana	3
Bok Choy and Tofu	5
Snack	3
3 servings Lemon-Rosemary White Bean Bruschetta	3
Dinner	8
Grilled Fish w/ Tartar Sauce	4
Crunchy Chocolate Mousse w/ Strawberries	4
Total Smart Points	**30**

DAY 8	
Breakfast	6
Mediterranean Strata w/ Goat Cheese	6
unsweetened fruit	0
Snack	13
5.5oz French fries (consume only half)	13
Lunch	6
Baked Pasta w/ Butternut Squash	6
Snack	
(other half of French fries)	
Dinner	5
Spinach and Feta Stuffed Chicken	4
Grilled Mango w/ Raspberry Granita	1
Total Smart Points	**30**

DAY 9	
Breakfast	4
Creamy Scrambled Eggs w/ Scallions	4
Cherries	0
Snack	4
Fruit Salad w/ Spiced Pistachio Yogurt	4
Lunch	5
Barley-Asparagus Risotto w/ Balsamic Vinegar	5
Snack	9
Maple Granola Bars	9
Dinner	8
BBQ Chicken Quesadilla	8
Total Smart Points	**30**

DAY 10	
Breakfast	6
Denver Omelette Mug	2
1 cup low-fat milk	4
Snack	8
1.6oz baked potato	5
1oz feta, crumbled	3

DAY 11	
Breakfast	8
2 tbsps. peanut butter	6
banana	0
1 slice bread	2
Snack	2
100-Calorie Beef Patties	2

DAY 12	
Breakfast	5
Mexican Breakfast Burritos	4
1 tbsp. guacamole	1
Snack	6
Italian Pepper and Egg Sandwich	6

Lunch	4
Bacon-Bundled BBQ Shrimp	4
Snack	4
Amazing Cheeseburger Patty	4
Dinner	8
Chinese Chicken Salad	5
Super Easy Chicken Noodle Soup	3
Total Smart Points	30

Lunch	7
Breaded Pork Cutlet	7
Garden Vegetable Soup	0
Snack	2
Denver Omelette in Mug	2
Dinner	11
lettuce, lemon juice w/	0
1 tbsp. olive oil	4
Grilled Salmon w/ Mustard	7
Total Smart Points	30

Lunch	5
Spice-Rubbed Pork Chops	5
Snack	4
1oz Colby cheese	4
Dinner	10
Grilled BBQ Tempeh	10
Total Smart Points	30

DAY 13	
Breakfast	6
Egg, Canadian Bacon, Avocado and Tomato	6
Mango	0
Snack	4
Strawberry and Blueberry Muffins	4
Lunch	9
Spicy BBQ Salmon and Veggies	9
Snack	4
Strawberry and Blueberry Muffins	4
Dinner	7
Roast Pork Dinner	7
Total Smart Points	30

DAY 14	
Breakfast	4
1 cup cooked oatmeal	1
berries	0
1 cup skim milk	3
Snack	4
Spicy Popcorn	4
Lunch	4
Chickpea and Brown Rice Veggie Burgers	4
Snack	4
2 servings Banana Chocolate-Chip Mini Muffins	4
Dinner	14
Steak and Mushrooms w/ Mashies	9
Ricotta & Almond Stuffed Dates	5
Total Smart Points	30

DAY 15	
Breakfast	9
1 slice American Cheese	4
1 small bagel	5
blackberries	0
Snack	4
1/4 cup almonds	4
Lunch	6
Filet Mignon w/ Red Wine Sauce	6
Snack	3
2 tbsps. Italian-type dressing	3
mixed greens	0
Dinner	8
Grilled Fish w/ Tartar Sauce	4
5oz white wine	4
Total Smart Points	30

DAY 16	
Breakfast	6

DAY 17	
Breakfast	6

DAY 18	
Breakfast	11

Fluffy Lemon-Ricotta Pancakes	6	Italian Pepper and Egg Sandwich	6	Quinoa and Apple Breakfast Cereal	6		
		pineapple	0	1 cup reduced-fat milk	5		
Snack	1	*Snack*	4	*Snack*	2		
Roasted Cauliflower w/ Lemon and Garlic	1	corn on a cob	4	Berry Bliss Ball	2		
Lunch	10	*Lunch*	5	*Lunch*	9		
lettuce, cucumber, and 1 tbsp. balsamic vinaigrette	1	Cellophane Noodles w/ Garlic, Cilantro and Cucumbers	5	Bacon Cheeseburger	5		
				Chili			
Cider-Glazed Pork Chops	9			Ultimate Fruit Salad	4		
Snack	4	*Snack*	4	*Snack*	2		
1oz tortilla chips	4	1/2 avocado	4	Berry Bliss Ball	2		
fat-free salsa	0						
Dinner	9	*Dinner*	11	*Dinner*	6		
Greek-Style Spaghetti Squash	2	Roasted Sirloin Beef (2 servings)	4	Tomato-Basil Sauce Eggplant Involtini (2 servings)	6		
Blueberry Pie	7	Blueberry Pie	7				
Total Smart Points	30	**Total Smart Points**	30	**Total Smart Points**	30		

DAY 19		**DAY 20**		**DAY 21**	
Breakfast	6	*Breakfast*	10	*Breakfast*	7
3oz tuna in water (can)	1	French Toast Nuggets	6	Oat and Apricot Bar	7
2 tbsps. ranch dressing	5	Grapefruit	0		
cucumber	0	1 tbsp. honey	4		
Snack	0	*Snack*	2	*Snack*	3
unsweetened fresh fruit	0	Greek-Style Spaghetti Squash	2	Buffalo Ranch Meatloaf	3
Lunch	11	*Lunch*	8	*Lunch*	5
1 cup cooked rice (white)	6	Artichoke and Red Pepper Frittata	5	Bacon Cheeseburger	5
Spicy Asian Pork Tenderloin	5			Chili	
		Apricot Quesadillas	3	watermelon	0
Snack	4	*Snack*	3	*Snack*	1
Coconut and Date Muesli Bar	4	1 cup fat-free Greek yogurt (plain)	3	1 cup cooked oatmeal	1
Dinner	9	*Dinner*	7	*Dinner*	14
Caramelized Onion and Mushroom Lasagna	9	Grilled Vegetables and Haloumi	7	Steak and Mushrooms w/ Mashies	9

				Chicken and Root Vegetable Soup	5
Total Smart Points	30	*Total Smart Points*	30	*Total Smart Points*	30

DAY 22		DAY 23		DAY 24	
Breakfast	6	*Breakfast*	6	*Breakfast*	5
Butternut Squash Fries	0	Cheesy Vegetable Sandwich	6	Fried Egg	3
Whole-Grain Banana Pancakes	6			Bacon Bundled Asparagus	2
Snack	4	*Snack*	0	*Snack*	2
Bacon-Bundled Shrimp	4	Butternut Squash Fries	0	Cauliflower, Mint, and Feta Fritters (2 servings)	2
Lunch	7	*Lunch*	10	*Lunch*	10
Kickin Chicken Pot Pie	7	Grilled BBQ Tempeh	10	Grilled Yellowfin Tuna w/ Teriyaki Sauce	6
				Crunchy Chocolate Mousse	4
Snack	0	*Snack*	5	*Snack*	1
berries	0	1 slice American Cheese	4	Cauliflower, Mint, and Feta Fritters	1
		Buffalo-Style Stuffed Celery	1		
Dinner	13	*Dinner*	9	*Dinner*	12
2 servings Amazing Cheeseburger Patty	8	Spicy BBQ Salmon and Veggies	9	2 servings Stir-Fry Beef and Broccoli	6
Peaches and Cream Tart	5			Baby Chocolate Butterfly Cakes (2 servings)	6
Total Smart Points	30	*Total Smart Points*	30	*Total Smart Points*	30

DAY 25		DAY 26		DAY 27	
Breakfast	4	*Breakfast*	4	*Breakfast*	7
2 servings Banana Chocolate Chips Mini Muffins	4	Bacon, Egg, and Spinach	4	Chicken BLT Sandwich	7
		strawberries	0	orange	0
Snack	3	*Snack*	0	*Snack*	6
3 servings Lemon-Rosemary White Bean	3	grapefruit	0	Cheesy Vegetable Sandwich	6
Lunch	8	*Lunch*	12	*Lunch*	7
Sesame-Ginger Pork Tenderloin	6	Beef, Mushroom and Barley Soup	6	Tomato-Basil Sauce Eggplant Involtini	3

Cream of Broccoli	2
Snack	4
Strawberry and Blueberry Muffins	4
Dinner	11
Grilled Salmon w/ Mustard	7
Spiced Turkish Mocha	4
Total Smart Points	30

Filet Mignon w/ Red Wine	6
Snack	2
100-Calorie Beef Patty	2
Dinner	12
Italian Pesto Chicken Burger	7
Ricotta and Almond Stuffed Dates	5
Total Smart Points	30

Ultimate Fruit Salad	4
Snack	0
banana	0
Dinner	10
2 servings Baked Chicken	4
Pulled Pork Special	6
Total Smart Points	30

DAY 28	
Breakfast	6
Cheesy Vegetable Sandwich	6
Snack	7
carrots	0
Italian-Pesto Chicken	7
Lunch	10
Taco-Stuffed Chicken	5
Chicken and Root Vegetable Soup	5
Snack	4
corn on a cob (medium)	4
Dinner	3
Grilled Trout w/ Stuffed Oregano and Lemon	3
Total Smart Points	30

DAY 29	
Breakfast	5
5 servings Mini Zucchini Quiche	5
Snack	4
1 slice American Cheese	4
grapes	0
Lunch	9
Caramelized Onion and Mushroom Lasagna	9
Snack	3
celery	0
1 tbsp. mayonnaise	3
Dinner	9
Tandoori Chicken w/ Chutney	7
Berry Bliss Ball	2
Total Smart Points	30

DAY 30	
Breakfast	3
green beans	0
3oz cooked pork chop	3
fat-free salsa	0
Snack	3
1 cup fat-free Greek yogurt (plain)	3
Lunch	9
Spicy BBQ Salmon and Veggies	9
Snack	4
Bacon-Bundled Shrimp	4
Dinner	11
Baked Vegetable Tart	9
Grilled Mango w/ Raspberry Granita (2 servings)	2
Total Smart Points	30

Month 2

DAY 1	
Breakfast	7
100-Calorie Beef Patties	2
hamburger bun	5
Snack	3
Buffalo-Style Stuffed Celery (3 servings)	3
Lunch	10
Breaded Pork Cutlet	7
Apricot Dessert Quesadillas	3
Snack	2
2 servings Roasted Cauliflower w/ Lemon	2
Dinner	8
Spinach and Feta Stuffed Chicken (2 servings)	8
nectarine	0
Total Smart Points	30

DAY 2	
Breakfast	7
1 tbsp. butter	5
1 slice bread	2
banana	0
Snack	7
Blueberry Pie	7
Lunch	8
BBQ Chicken Quesadilla	8
blackberries	0
Snack	3
Sultana Apple Slice	3
Dinner	5
Spicy Asian Pork Tenderloin	5
Total Smart Points	30

DAY 3	
Breakfast	10
Maple Granola Bars	9
1 cup unsweetened almond milk	1
Snack	0
apple	0
Lunch	5
Spice-Rubbed Pork Chops	5
Snack	9
Maple Granola Bar	9
Dinner	6
Sesame-Ginger Pork Tenderloin	6
Total Smart Points	30

DAY 4	
Breakfast	13
Hash and Eggs	8
3 slices cooked bacon	5
Snack	3
Baby Chocolate Butterfly Cakes	3
Lunch	6
Pork Tenderloin Roast (2 servings)	6
Snack	3
Baby Chocolate Butterfly Cakes	3

DAY 5	
Breakfast	5
Denver Omelette in Mug	2
1oz feta, crumbled	3
Snack	3
celery	0
1 tablespoon mayo	3
Lunch	7
Grilled Salmon w/ Mustard	7
Snack	7
1 tbsp. butter	5
1 slice bread	2

DAY 6	
Breakfast	4
Passion Fruit Soufflé	4
blueberries	0
Snack	4
1/2 cup mashed potatoes	4
Lunch	8
Bacon-Bundled BBQ Shrimp (2 servings)	8
Snack	4
4 tbsps. cream, half and half	4
cantaloupe	0

Dinner	5
Bacon Cheeseburger	5
Chili	
Total Smart Points	**30**

Dinner	8
6oz cooked skinless chicken breast	4
fat-free salsa	0
Spiced Turkish Mocha	4
Total Smart Points	**30**

Dinner	10
Seasoned Pork Tenderloin	4
1 cup cooked rice (white)	6
Total Smart Points	**30**

DAY 7	
Breakfast	5
Steak and Eggs	5
green beans	0
Snack	4
1 medium corn on the cob	4
Lunch	7
Grilled Vegetables and Haloumi	7
Snack	4
2oz Deli sliced turkey	1
1oz Feta, crumbled	3
Dinner	10
Bacon Cheeseburger Chili	5
Ricotta and Almond Stuffed Dates	5
Total Smart Points	**30**

DAY 8	
Breakfast	10
2 scrambled eggs with milk and butter	6
English Muffin	4
Snack	1
Roasted Cauliflower w/ Lemon and Garlic	1
Lunch	4
Grilled Fish w/ Tartar Sauce	4
Snack	6
1oz Colby cheese	4
3oz cooked Chicken breast, skinless	2
Dinner	9
Caramelized Onion and Mushroom Lasagna	9
Total Smart Points	**30**

DAY 9	
Breakfast	4
Bacon, Egg, and Spinach	4
mixed berries	0
Snack	4
Spicy Popcorn	4
Lunch	7
Tandoori Chicken w/ Chutney	7
Snack	4
1 medium corn on the cob	4
Dinner	11
Grilled Vegetables and Haloumi	7
Spiced Turkish Mocha	4
Total Smart Points	**30**

DAY 10	
Breakfast	2
Denver Omelette in Mug	2
pineapple	0
Snack	0
berries	0
Lunch	11

DAY 11	
Breakfast	7
Chicken BLT Sandwich	7
Snack	3
1/2 cup cooked sweet potatoes	3
Lunch	4

DAY 12	
Breakfast	4
Mexican Breakfast Burritos	4
Snack	4
3oz cooked ground beef	4
lettuce	0
Lunch	15

Pulled Pork Special	6
2oz plain hamburger bun	5
Snack	**4**
Bacon Bundled Asparagus (2 servings)	4
Dinner	**13**
Roast Pork Dinner	7
Beef, Mushroom and Barley Soup	6
Total Smart Points	**30**

Amazing Cheeseburger Patty	4
Snack	**4**
Strawberry and Blueberry Muffins	4
Dinner	**12**
BBQ Chicken Quesadilla	8
1/2 cup mashed potatoes	4
Total Smart Points	**30**

100-Calorie Beef Patties	2
5.5oz French fries	13
Snack	**3**
Baby Chocolate Butterfly Cakes	3
Dinner	**4**
Spinach and Feta Stuffed Chicken	4
Total Smart Points	**30**

DAY 13	
Breakfast	**9**
Italian Pepper and Egg Sandwich	6
1 cup Greek yogurt plain	3
Snack	**3**
Cauliflower, Mint and Feta Fritters (3 servings)	3
Lunch	**6**
Roasted Salmon in Honey-Mustard	6
Snack	**3**
Garden Vegetable Soup	0
3 slices cooked turkey	3
Dinner	**9**
Cider-Glazed Pork Chops	9
Total Smart Points	**30**

DAY 14	
Breakfast	**6**
Fluffy Lemon-Ricotta Pancakes	6
Raspberries	0
Snack	**3**
3 slices cooked turkey Bacon	3
Lunch	**3**
Grilled Trout w/ Stuffed Oregano and Lemon	3
Snack	**4**
1/4 cup almonds	4
Dinner	**14**
Grilled BBQ Tempeh	10
Ultimate Fruit Salad	4
Total Smart Points	**30**

DAY 15	
Breakfast	**6**
Whole-Grain Banana Pancakes	6
Snack	**6**
banana	0
2 tbsps. peanut butter	6
Lunch	**8**
Roasted Sirloin Beef	2
1 cup cooked white rice	6
Snack	**1**
Roasted Cauliflower w/ Lemon and Garlic	1
fresh fruit	0
Dinner	**9**
Spicy BBQ Salmon w/ Mustard	9
Veggie Soup	0
Total Smart Points	**30**

DAY 16	
Breakfast	**6**

DAY 17	
Breakfast	**8**

DAY 18	
Breakfast	**7**

Mediterranean Strata w/ Goat Cheese	6
Snack	*4*
Coconut and Date Muesli Bar	4
Lunch	*5*
Artichoke and Red Pepper Frittata	5
Snack	*1*
1 cup cooked oatmeal	1
berries	0
Dinner	*14*
Artichoke and Red Pepper Frittata	5
Cream of Broccoli	2
Blueberry Pie	7
Total Smart Points	**30**

Hash and Eggs	8
orange	0
Snack	*4*
California Club Wrap	4
Lunch	*6*
Baked Pasta w/ Butternut Squash	6
Snack	*1*
Lemon-Rosemary White Bean Bruschetta	1
banana	0
Dinner	*11*
Filet Mignon w/ Red Wine Sauce	6
5oz red wine	5
Total Smart Points	**30**

3 slices cooked turkey bacon	3
1oz cheddar cheese	4
Snack	*1*
3oz cooked shrimp	1
Lunch	*9*
Caramelized Onion and Mushroom Lasagna	9
Snack	*2*
Berry Bliss Balls	2
Dinner	*11*
Kickin Chicken Pot Pie	7
Italian-Inspired Vegetable Soup	0
Spiced Turkish Mocha	4
Total Smart Points	**30**

DAY 19	
Breakfast	*11*
Chocolate-Banana Mini Muffins (2 servings)	4
1 cup whole milk	7
Snack	*3*
Lemon-Rosemary Bean Bruschetta (3 servings)	3
Lunch	*6*
Stir-fry Beef & Broccoli (2 servings)	6
Snack	*1*
Buffalo-Style Stuffed Celery	1
Dinner	*9*
Eggplant Parmigiana (2 servings)	6

DAY 20	
Breakfast	*4*
Creamy Scrambled Eggs w/ Scallions	4
Snack	*4*
Bacon Bundled Asparagus (2 servings)	4
Lunch	*5*
Barley-Asparagus Risotto w/ Balsamic Vinegar	5
Snack	*8*
Strawberry and Blueberry Muffins (2 servings)	8
Dinner	*9*
Tomato-Basil Sauce Eggplant Involtini	6

DAY 21	
Breakfast	*6*
Cheesy Vegetable Sandwich	6
Snack	*1*
Roasted Cauliflower w/ Lemon and Garlic	1
Lunch	*9*
Baked Vegetable Tart	9
Snack	*9*
2oz plain hamburger bun	5
Amazing Cheeseburger Patty	4
Dinner	*5*
Bok Choy and Tofu Stir-Fry	5

Super Easy Chicken Noodle Soup	3	
Total Smart Points	30	

(2 servings)		
Sultana Apple Slice	3	
Total Smart Points	30	

Total Smart Points	30	

DAY 22

Breakfast	7
1 cup fat-free cottage cheese	2
1 small bagel	5
Snack	5
Chinese Chicken Salad	5
Lunch	5
Cellophane Noodles w/ Garlic, Cilantro and Cucumbers	5
Snack	0
Garden Vegetable Soup	0
banana	0
Dinner	13
Sesame-Ginger Pork Tenderloin	6
Blueberry Pie	7
Total Smart Points	30

DAY 23

Breakfast	9
Steak and Eggs	5
1oz Colby cheese	4
Snack	4
California Club Wrap	4
Lunch	4
Chickpea and Brown Rice Veggie Burgers	4
Snack	4
Berry Bliss Balls (2 servings)	4
Dinner	9
Caramelized Onion and Mushroom Lasagna	9
Total Smart Points	30

DAY 24

Breakfast	6
Quinoa and Apple Breakfast Cereal	6
Snack	4
1oz tortilla chips	4
fat-free salsa	0
Lunch	4
Fajita-Stuffed Chicken	4
Fresh Vegetable Soup	0
Snack	4
Spicy Popcorn	4
Dinner	12
Breaded Pork Cutlet	7
Chicken and Root Vegetable Soup	5
Total Smart Points	30

DAY 25

Breakfast	6
French Toast Nuggets	6
Snack	4
Fruit Salad w/ Spiced Pistachio Yogurt	4
Lunch	6
Taco-Stuffed Chicken	5
Grilled Mango w/ Raspberry Granita	1

DAY 26

Breakfast	8
Cheesy and Saucy Egg Sandwich	8
Snack	1
Butternut Squash Fries	0
3oz tuna in water (can)	1
Lunch	4
California Club Wrap	4

DAY 27

Breakfast	7
Oat and Apricot Bar	7
Snack	0
mixed berries	0
Lunch	13
General Tso's Chicken	8
Ricotta and Almond Stuffed Dates	5

	Snack	4
	Coconut and Date Muesli Bar	4
	Dinner	**10**
	Feta-Stuffed Chicken Burgers	6
	Crunchy Chocolate Mousse w/ Strawberries	4
	Total Smart Points	**30**

	Snack	4
	Strawberry and Blueberry Muffins	4
	Dinner	**13**
	Roast Pork Dinner	7
	Beef, Mushroom and Barley Soup	6
	Total Smart Points	**30**

	Snack	0
	baby carrots	0
	Dinner	**10**
	Bacon Cheeseburger	5
	Chili	
	Bok Choy and Tofu Stir-Fry	5
	Total Smart Points	**30**

DAY 28	
Breakfast	**6**
Egg, Canadian Bacon, Avocado, and Tomato	6
Snack	**7**
3oz tuna in water (can)	1
2 tbsps. mayonnaise	6
Lunch	**5**
Cellophane Noodles w/ Garlic, Cilantro and Cucumbers	5
Snack	**0**
Butternut Squash Fries	0
Pepper and Mushroom Kebabs w/ Dip	0
Dinner	**12**
Italian Pesto Chicken Burger	7
Chicken and Root Vegetable Soup	5
Total Smart Points	**30**

DAY 29	
Breakfast	**3**
Mini Zucchini Quiche (3 servings)	3
Snack	**9**
1.6oz plain baked potato	5
1oz cheddar or Colby	4
Lunch	**5**
Baked Chicken	2
Super Easy Chicken Noodle Soup	3
Snack	**0**
grapes	0
Dinner	**13**
Grilled Yellowfin Tuna w/ Teriyaki Sauce	6
Blueberry Pie	7
Total Smart Points	**30**

DAY 30	
Breakfast	**8**
Hash and Eggs	8
fresh fruit	0
Snack	**4**
Amazing Cheeseburger Patty	4
Lunch	**6**
Greek-Style Spaghetti Squash	2
Ultimate Fruit Salad	4
Snack	**3**
3 slices cooked turkey	3
lettuce	0
Dinner	**9**
Steak and Mushrooms w/ Mashies	9
Total Smart Points	**30**

Month 3

DAY 1	DAY 2	DAY 3

Breakfast	7
1 cup fat-free cottage cheese	2
1 small bagel	5
Snack	**0**
apple	0
Lunch	**6**
Pulled Pork Special	6
Snack	**6**
2 tbsps. peanut butter	6
banana	0
Dinner	**11**
Kickin Chicken Pot Pie	7
Strawberry and Blueberry Muffins	4
Total Smart Points	**30**

Breakfast	6
2 scrambled eggs with milk and butter	6
banana	0
Snack	**0**
Pepper and Mushroom Kebabs w/ Dip	0
Lunch	**12**
Pork Tenderloin Roast (2 servings)	6
1 cup cooked white rice	6
Snack	**0**
Garden Vegetable Soup	0
Dinner	**12**
Grilled BBQ Tempeh	10
Cream of Broccoli	2
Total Smart Points	**30**

Breakfast	9
Steak and Eggs	5
1oz cheddar cheese	4
Snack	**4**
Bacon-Bundled BBQ Shrimp	4
Lunch	**8**
General Tso's Chicken	8
Snack	**3**
Sultana Apple Slice	3
Dinner	**6**
Grilled Yellowfin Tuna w/ Teriyaki Sauce	6
Total Smart Points	**30**

DAY 4	
Breakfast	**7**
Steak and Eggs	5
mixed berries	0
1 slice bread	2
Snack	**2**
Bacon Bundled Asparagus	2
Lunch	**8**
Roasted Sirloin Beef	2
1 cup cooked white rice	6
Snack	**1**
Lemon-Rosemary White Bean Bruschetta	1
Dinner	**12**
Breaded Pork Cutlet	7

DAY 5	
Breakfast	**6**
Quinoa and Apple Breakfast Cereal	6
Snack	**4**
Spicy Popcorn	4
Lunch	**4**
Grilled Fish w/ Tartar Sauce	4
Snack	**9**
Maple Granola Bar	9
Dinner	**7**
Eggplant Parmigiana	6

DAY 6	
Breakfast	**8**
Cheesy and Saucy Egg Sandwich	8
Snack	**4**
Chocolate-Banana Mini Muffins (2 servings)	4
Lunch	**3**
Stir-fry Beef & Broc	3
Italian-Inspired Vegetable Soup	0
Snack	**7**
Blueberry Pie	7
Dinner	**8**
Amazing Cheeseburger	8

Chicken and Root Vegetable Soup	5
Total Smart Points	**30**

(2 servings)	
Grilled Mango w/ Raspberry Granita	1
Total Smart Points	**30**

Patty (2 servings)	
Fresh Vegetable Soup	0
Total Smart Points	**30**

DAY 7	
Breakfast	6
Whole-Grain Banana Pancakes	6
Snack	6
2 tbsps. mayonnaise	6
mixed greens	0
Lunch	5
Spice-Rubbed Pork Chops	5
Snack	3
Baby Chocolate Butterfly Cakes	3
Dinner	10
Barley-Asparagus Risotto w/ Balsamic Vinegar	5
Peaches and Cream Tart	5
Total Smart Points	**30**

DAY 8	
Breakfast	5
Fried Egg	3
Bacon Bundled Asparagus	2
Snack	6
banana	0
2 tbsps. peanut butter	6
Lunch	3
Grilled Trout w/ Stuffed Oregano and Lemon	3
Snack	6
3oz tuna in water (can)	1
2 tbsps. ranch dressing	5
lettuce	0
Dinner	10
California Club Wrap	4
4 tbsps. Italian-type dressing	6
lettuce, cucumber	0
Total Smart Points	**30**

DAY 9	
Breakfast	5
Coconut and Date Muesli Bar	4
1 cup almond milk	1
Snack	4
1/4 cup almonds	4
Mixed berries	0
Lunch	6
Greek-Style Spaghetti Squash	2
Spiced Turkish Mocha	4
Snack	6
Mexican Breakfast Burritos	4
2 tbsps. guacamole	2
Dinner	9
Filet Mignon w/ Red Wine Sauce	6
Apricot Dessert Quesadillas	3
Total Smart Points	**30**

DAY 10	
Breakfast	10
1 tbsp. butter	5
1 small Bagel	5
Snack	2
Berry Bliss Balls	2
Lunch	11
Spicy Asian Pork	5

DAY 11	
Breakfast	7
Oat and Apricot Bar	7
Snack	3
Cauliflower, Mint and Feta Fritters (3 servings)	3
Lunch	9
Buffalo Ranch Meatloaf	3

DAY 12	
Breakfast	6
Egg, Canadian Bacon, Avocado, and Tomato	6
Snack	2
Berry Bliss Balls	2
Lunch	4
Spinach and Feta Stuffed	4

Tenderloin	
1 cup cooked brown rice	6
Snack	**0**
Zero Hero Soup	0
Dinner	**7**
Chickpea and Brown Rice Veggie Burgers	4
Super Easy Chicken Noodle Soup	3
Total Smart Points	**30**

Beef, Mushroom and Barley Soup	6
Snack	**4**
1 cup cooked oatmeal	1
1/2 cup low-fat 1% milk	2
1 tsp white sugar	1
Dinner	**7**
Fajita-Stuffed Chicken	4
Garden Vegetable Soup	0
3 slices cooked turkey	3
Total Smart Points	**30**

Chicken	
Snack	**8**
Amazing Cheeseburger Patty	4
1oz Colby cheese	4
Dinner	**10**
Roasted Salmon in Honey-Mustard	6
Ultimate Fruit Salad	4
Total Smart Points	**30**

DAY 13

Breakfast	**6**
Cheesy Vegetable Sandwich	6
Snack	**2**
hardboiled egg	2
Lunch	**9**
Baked Vegetable Tart	9
Snack	**3**
Bacon Bundled Asparagus	2
2 tbsps. low-fat cheddar cheese (shredded)	1
Dinner	**10**
Bacon Cheeseburger Chili	5
Ricotta and Almond Stuffed Dates	5
Total Smart Points	**30**

DAY 14

Breakfast	**10**
French Toast Nuggets	6
1 tbsp. honey	4
Snack	**4**
corn on a cob	4
Lunch	**4**
100-Calorie Beef Patties (2 servings)	4
Snack	**5**
Buffalo-Style Stuffed Celery (5 servings)	5
Dinner	**7**
Seasoned Pork Tenderloin	4
1/2 cup cooked white rice	3
Total Smart Points	**30**

DAY 15

Breakfast	**6**
Mediterranean Strata w/ Goat Cheese	6
Snack	**2**
3oz cooked Chicken breast, skinless	2
Lunch	**7**
Tandoori Chicken w/ Chutney	7
Snack	**6**
4 tbsps. Italian-type dressing	6
lettuce	0
Dinner	**9**
Chinese Chicken Salad	5
Fruit Salad w/ Spiced Pistachio Yogurt	4
Total Smart Points	**30**

DAY 16

Breakfast	**7**
1 English Muffin	4

DAY 17

Breakfast	**5**
Mexican Breakfast	4

DAY 18

Breakfast	**4**
1 cup cooked oatmeal	1

1oz crumbled feta	3
mixed berries	0
Snack	
Butternut Squash Fries	0
Lunch	9
Spicy BBQ Salmon w/ Mustard	9
Snack	5
1/2 cup mashed potatoes	4
2oz Deli sliced turkey	1
Dinner	9
Caramelized Onion and Mushroom Lasagna	9
Total Smart Points	30

Burritos	
1 tbsps. guacamole	1
Snack	8
2oz tortilla chips	8
fat-free salsa	0
Lunch	7
Roast Pork Dinner	7
Snack	1
Roasted Cauliflower w/ Lemon and Garlic	1
Dinner	9
Cider-Glazed Pork Chops	9
Total Smart Points	30

1 cup skim milk	3
mixed berries	0
Snack	5
Ricotta and Almond Stuffed Dates	5
Lunch	7
Grilled Vegetables and Haloumi	7
Snack	2
lettuce, cucumber, and	0
2 tbsps. balsamic vinaigrette	2
Dinner	12
BBQ Chicken Quesadilla	8
Veggie Soup	0
Crunchy Chocolate Mousse w/ Strawberries	4
Total Smart Points	30

DAY 19	
Breakfast	6
Egg, Canadian Bacon, Avocado and Tomato	6
Mango	0
Snack	7
1 tbsp. butter	5
1 slice bread	2
Lunch	2
Baked Chicken	2
Snack	6
1 cup cooked sweet potatoes	6
Dinner	9
Grilled Salmon w/ Mustard	7
Chocolate-Banana Mini	2

DAY 20	
Breakfast	6
Fluffy Lemon-Ricotta Pancakes	6
Snack	13
5.5oz French fries (consume half only)	13
Lunch	5
Artichoke and Red Pepper Frittata	5
Snack	
(the remaining half of French fries)	
Dinner	6
Feta-Stuffed Chicken Burgers	6

DAY 21	
Breakfast	9
Chicken BLT Sandwich	7
1/4 avocado	2
Snack	4
2oz Deli sliced turkey	1
1oz Feta, crumbled	3
Lunch	6
Sesame-Ginger Pork Tenderloin	6
Snack	2
Cauliflower, Mint and Feta Fritters (2 servings)	2
Dinner	9
Italian Pesto Chicken Burger	7
Cream of Broccoli	2

Muffins	
Total Smart Points	30

Total Smart Points	30

Total Smart Points	30

DAY 22	
Breakfast	6
Italian Pepper and Egg Sandwich	6
Snack	6
Cheesy Vegetable Sandwich	6
Lunch	5
Taco-Stuffed Chicken	5
fat-free salsa	0
Snack	5
6oz cooked shrimp	2
1 tbsp. mayonnaise	3
Dinner	8
Bok Choy and Tofu Stir-Fry	5
Sultana Apple Slice	3
Total Smart Points	30

DAY 23	
Breakfast	8
3 slices bacon	5
1 fried egg	3
orange	0
Snack	10
2oz tortilla chips	8
2 tbsps. guacamole	2
Lunch	3
Tomato-Basil Sauce Eggplant Involtini	3
Snack	0
mixed berries	0
Dinner	9
Steak and Mushrooms w/ Mashies	9
Total Smart Points	30

DAY 24	
Breakfast	8
Cheesy and Saucy Egg Sandwich	8
grapes	0
Snack	
Lunch	5
Cellophane Noodles w/ Garlic, Cilantro and Cucumbers	5
Snack	4
1/4 cup almonds	4
Dinner	13
Baked Pasta w/ Butternut Squash	6
Blueberry Pie	7
Total Smart Points	30

DAY 25	
Breakfast	11
Chocolate-Banana Mini Muffins (2 servings)	4
1 cup whole milk	7
Snack	5
Chicken and Root Vegetable Soup	5
Lunch	5
Bacon Cheeseburger Chili	5
Snack	4

DAY 26	
Breakfast	8
Bacon-Bundled BBQ Shrimp (2 servings)	8
pineapple	0
Snack	4
1/2 cup mashed potatoes	4
Lunch	9
Caramelized Onion and Mushroom Lasagna	9
Snack	2

DAY 27	
Breakfast	6
Feta-Stuffed Chicken Burgers	6
blueberries	0
Snack	0
Garden Vegetable Soup	0
banana	0
Lunch	6
Roasted Salmon in Honey-Mustard	6
Snack	12

4 tbsps. cream, half and half	4
cantaloupe	0
Dinner	**5**
Spice-Rubbed Pork Chops	5
Total Smart Points	**30**

Chocolate-Banana Mini Muffins (2 servings)	2
Dinner	**7**
Grilled Vegetables and Haloumi	7
Total Smart Points	**30**

1 cup fat-free cottage cheese	2
2 small bagels	10
Dinner	**6**
Sesame-Ginger Pork Tenderloin	6
Total Smart Points	**30**

DAY 28	
Breakfast	**10**
Maple Granola Bars	9
1 cup unsweetened almond milk	1
Snack	**1**
Roasted Cauliflower w/ Lemon and Garlic	1
Lunch	**7**
Italian Pesto Chicken Burger	7
Snack	**4**
2oz Deli sliced turkey	1
1oz Feta, crumbled	3
Dinner	**8**
Spinach and Feta Stuffed Chicken	4
Fruit Salad w/ Spiced Pistachio Yogurt	4
Total Smart Points	**30**

DAY 29	
Breakfast	**10**
2 scrambled eggs with milk and butter	6
English Muffin	4
Snack	**3**
Sultana Apple Slice	3
Lunch	**8**
BBQ Chicken Quesadilla	8
Fresh Vegetable Soup	0
Snack	**0**
Butternut Squash Fries	0
Dinner	**9**
Spicy BBQ Salmon w/ Mustard	9
Total Smart Points	**30**

DAY 30	
Breakfast	**8**
Cheesy and Saucy Egg Sandwich	8
cantaloupe	0
Snack	**4**
Coconut and Date Muesli Bar	4
Lunch	**5**
Barley-Asparagus Risotto w/ Balsamic Vinegar	5
Snack	**0**
mango	0
Dinner	**13**
Baked Vegetable Tart	9
Crunchy Chocolate Mousse w/ Strawberries	4
Total Smart Points	**30**

Conclusion

By now, you must have a good understanding of how the Weight Watchers program works, and come up with your own meal plans. You have a lot of recipes that you can mix and match plus the tools that can help you determine the right Smart Points value.

If you enjoyed this book, please take the time to leave me a review on Amazon. I appreciate your honest feedback, and it really helps me to continue producing high-quality books.

Made in the USA
San Bernardino, CA
08 January 2018